The Essential Guide to Nursing Practice

Applying ANA's Scope AND Standards IN Practice AND Education

EDITORS: **Kathleen M. White,** PhD, RN, NEA-BC, FAAN
Ann O'Sullivan, MSN, RN, NE-BC, CNE

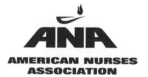

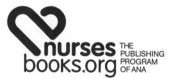

American Nurses Association
Silver Spring, MD
2012

Library of Congress Cataloging-in-Publication data

The essential guide to nursing practice : applying ANA's scope and standards to practice and education / Kathleen M. White, Ann O'Sullivan, editors.
    p. ; cm.
    Includes bibliographical references and index.
    ISBN 978-1-55810-458-7 (softcover / pbk. : alk. paper) — ISBN 978-1-55810-455-6 (ebook, PDF format) — ISBN 978-1-55810-456-3 (ebook, EPUB format) — ISBN 978-1-55810-457-0 (ebook, Mobipocket format)
    I. White, Kathleen M. (Kathleen Murphy), 1953- II. O'Sullivan, Ann, RN. III. American Nurses Association. IV. American Nurses Association. Nursing : scope and standards of practice. V. American Nurses Association. Nursing's social policy statement.
    [DNLM: 1. Nursing--standards—United States. 2. Clinical Competence--United States. 3. Nurse's Role—United States. WY 16 AA1]

    610.73—dc23

2012019791

The American Nurses Association (ANA) is a national professional association. This ANA publication—*The Essential Guide to Nursing Practice: Applying ANA's Scope and Standards in Practice and Education*—reflects the thinking of the nursing profession on various issues and should be reviewed in conjunction with state board of nursing policies and practices. State law, rules, and regulations govern the practice of nursing, while *The Essential Guide to Nursing Practice: Applying ANA's Scope and Standards in Practice and Education* guides nurses in the application of their professional skills and responsibilities.

American Nurses Association
8515 Georgia Avenue, Suite 400
Silver Spring, MD 20910-3492
1-800-274-4ANA
http://www.NursingWorld.org

Published by Nursesbooks.org
The Publishing Program of ANA
http://www.Nursesbooks.org/

    ISBN-13: 978-1-55810-458-7   SAN: 851-3481   5K   06/2012
    First printing: June 2012

Contents

Contributors   xi

Introduction   xiv
      Kathleen M. White, PhD, RN, NEA-BC, FAAN and
      Ann O'Sullivan, MSN, RN, NE-BC, CNE

Chapter 1—Nursing's Social Policy Statement   1
      Catherine E. Neuman, MSN, RN, NEA-BC

Overview   1
    Social Context of Nursing   1
    Definition of Nursing   4
    Knowledge Base for Nursing Practice   5
    Regulation of Nursing Practice   6
Use of the Social Policy Statement in Practice   7
Conclusion   8
Discussion Topics   9
References and Other Sources   9

Chapter 2—Scope of Nursing Practice   11
      Ann O'Sullivan, MSN, RN, CNE, NE-BC

Overview of Scope of Nursing Practice   11
    Nursing Process   12
Characteristics of Nursing Practice   13
Model of Professional Nursing Practice Regulation   14
    Nurse Practice Acts   15
    Institutional Policies and Procedures   16
    Self-Determination   17
Conclusion   19
Exercises for Application   19
References and Other Sources   21

Chapter 3—Standards of Nursing Practice   **23**
         Kathleen M. White, PhD, RN, NEA-BC, FAAN
   Nursing as a Profession   23
   Standards of Professional Nursing Practice   24
   Application of the Standards in Nursing Practice   26
     Education   27
     Administration   28
     Performance and Quality Improvement   29
     Research   30
   Key Legal and Practical Implications of Standards   30
     Nursing Specialty Practice   31
     ANA Recognition of Specialty   32
   Conclusion   33
   Discussion Topics   33
   References and Other Sources   33

Chapter 4—Standard 1. Assessment   **35**
         Sharon J. Olsen, PhD, RN, AOCN
   Definition and Explanation of the Standard   35
     Data Collection   35
     Synthesis   37
   Application of the Standard in Practice   38
     Education   38
     Administration   39
     Performance and Quality Improvement   39
     Research   40
   Conclusion   41
   Case Study and Discussion Topics   41
   References and Other Sources   43

Chapter 5—Standard 2. Diagnosis   **45**
         Julie Stanik-Hutt, PhD, ACNP-BC, CCNS, FAAN
   Definition and Explanation of the Standard   45
     Types of Diagnoses Used in Nursing   46
     The Diagnostic Process   48
   Application of the Standard in Practice   52
     Education   52
     Administration   53

Performance and Quality Improvement   53

    Research   54

Conclusion   54

Case Studies and Discussion Topics   55

References and Other Sources   58

Chapter 6—Standard 3. Outcomes Identification   **63**

Margaret G. Williams, PhD, RN, CNE, and
Kathleen M. White, PhD, RN, NEA-BC, FAAN

Definition and Explanation of the Standard   63

    Structure, Process, and Outcomes Model   66

    Nursing Outcomes Classification   66

    Omaha System   67

    Some Characteristics of Outcome Identification   68

Application of the Standard in Practice   68

    Education   68

    Administration   69

    Performance and Quality Improvement   70

    Research   70

Conclusion   71

Case Study   71

    Scenario Based on Person with Congestive Heart Failure   71

    Learning Objectives   71

References and Other Sources   73

Chapter 7—Standard 4. Planning   **75**

Jennifer Matthews, PhD, RN, ACNS-BC, CNE, FAAN

Definition and Explanation of the Standard   75

Application of the Standard in Practice   79

    Education   79

    Administration   79

    Performance and Quality Improvement   79

    Research   80

Conclusion   81

Case Study with Discussion Topics   81

References and Other Sources   84

Chapter 8—Standard 5. Implementation   **87**
         Beth Martin, MSN, RN, CCNS, ACNP-BC, ACHPN
    Definition and Explanation of the Standard   87
       Standard 5A. Coordination of Care   94
       Standard 5B. Health Teaching and Health Promotion   94
       Standard 5C. Consultation   95
       Standard 5D. Prescriptive Authority and Treatment   95
    Application of the Standard in Practice   96
       Education   96
       Administration   96
       Research   97
       Performance and Quality Improvement   98
    Conclusion   98
    Case Study with Discussion Topics   99
    References and Other Sources   101

Chapter 9—Standard 6. Evaluation   **105**
         Janet Y. Harris, MSN, RN, CNAA-BC, and
         Kim W. Hoover, PhD, RN
    Definition and Explanation of the Standard   105
    Application of the Standard in Practice   106
       Education   106
       Administration   107
       Performance and Quality Improvement   108
       Research   109
    Conclusion   109
    Case Studies and Discussion Topics   110
    References and Other Sources   110

Chapter 10—Standard 7. Ethics   **113**
         Linda L. Olson, PhD, RN, NEA-BC
    Definition and Explanation of the Standard   113
    Application of the Standard in Practice   115
       Education   115
       Administration   116
       Performance and Quality Improvement   117
       Research   118
    Conclusion   118

Case Study and Discussion Topics   119
References and Other Sources   121

Chapter 11—Standard 8. Education   **123**
     Pamela A. Kulbok, DNSc, RN, PHCNS-BC, FAAN
Definition and Explanation of the Standard   123
Application of the Standard in Practice   125
    Education   125
    Administration   126
    Performance and Quality Improvement   127
    Research   128
Conclusion   128
Case Study and Discussion Topics   129
References and Other Sources   130

Chapter 12—Standard 9. Evidence-Based Practice and Research   **133**
     Kathleen M. White, PhD, RN, NEA-BC, FAAN
Definition and Explanation of the Standard   133
Application of the Standard in Practice   135
    Education   135
    Administration   136
    Performance and Quality Improvement   137
    Research   137
Conclusion   138
Case Study and Discussion Topics   138
Online Resources   141
    Cumulative Index to Nursing and Allied Health Literature
      (CINAHL®)   141
    Cochrane Library   141
    Database of Abstracts of Reviews of Effects (DARE)   141
    Google Scholar   141
    Joanna Briggs Institute (JBI)   142
    National Guideline Clearinghouse (NGC)   142
    PubMed/MEDLINE   142
    Trip Database—Clinical Search Engine (Trip)   142
    SUMSearch   142
    Virginia Henderson International Nursing Library (VHINL)
      Database   143
References and Other Sources   143

Chapter 13—Standard 10. Quality of Practice   **145**
Brenda L. Lyon, PhD, CNS, FAAN
Definition and Explanation of the Standard   145
Application of the Standard in Practice   147
  Education   147
  Administration   148
  Performance and Quality Improvement   148
  Research   149
Conclusion   149
Case Study and Discussion Topics   150
References and Other Sources   150

Chapter 14—Standard 11. Communication   **153**
Ann O'Sullivan, MS, RN, CNE, NE-BC
Definition and Explanation of the Standard   153
Application of the Standard in Practice   156
  Education   156
  Administration   157
  Performance and Quality Improvement   158
  Research   159
Conclusion   159
Case Studies and Discussion Topics   160
References and Other Sources   160

Chapter 15—Standard 12. Leadership   **163**
Mary-Anne D. Ponti, MS, RN, MBA, CNAA-BC, FACHE
Definition and Explanation of the Standard   163
Application of the Standard in Practice   166
  Education   166
  Administration   167
  Performance and Quality Improvement   167
  Research   168
Conclusion   169
Case Studies and Discussion Topics   169
References and Other Sources   171

Chapter 16—Standard 13. Collaboration   **173**
Pamela Brown, PhD, RN
Definition and Explanation of the Standard   173

The Essential Guide to Nursing Practice

Application of the Standard in Practice   176
    Education   176
    Administration   177
    Performance and Quality Improvement   179
    Research   179
Conclusion   181
Case Studies and Discussion Topics   181
References and Other Sources   183

Chapter 17—Standard 14. Professional Practice Evaluation   **187**
    Joanne V. Hickey, PhD, RN, ACNP-BC, FAAN
Definition and Explanation of the Standard   187
Application of the Standard in Practice   188
    Education   188
    Administration   189
    Performance and Quality Improvement   190
    Research   190
Conclusion   191
Case Studies and Discussion Topics   191
References   192

Chapter 18—Standard 15. Resource Utilization   **193**
    Kathleen M. White, PhD, RN, NEA-BC, FAAN
Definition and Explanation of the Standard   193
Application of the Standard in Practice   195
    Education   195
    Administration   196
    Performance and Quality Improvement   196
    Research   196
Conclusion   197
Case Study and Discussion Topics   197
    Case Study   197
    Discussion Topics: Initial   198
    Discussion Topics: Follow-Up   198
References and Other Sources   198

Chapter 19—Standard 16. Environmental Health   **201**
    Karen Ballard, RN, MA, FAAN
Definition and Explanation of the Standard   201

Application of the Standard in Practice   204

    Education   204

    Administration   205

    Performance and Quality Improvement   206

    Research   207

Conclusion   207

Case Studies and Discussion Topics   207

    Case Study 1. Workplace Noise   207

    Discussion Topics   208

    Example for Solution and Discussion   208

    Case Study 2. A Unit Green Team   209

    Discussion Topics   209

    Example for Solution and Discussion   210

Online Resources   210

References and Other Sources   211

Index   **215**

Contributors

Editors and Authors

Kathleen M. White, PhD, RN, NEA-BC, FAAN

Associate Professor, Johns Hopkins School of Nursing, Department of Health Systems and Outcomes; Clinical Nurse Specialist, The Johns Hopkins Hospital

Ann O'Sullivan, MSN, RN, CNE, NE-BC

Assistant Dean, Associate Professor, Blessing-Rieman College of Nursing

Authors

Karen A. Ballard, MA, RN, FAAN
  Nursing Consultant
  Nursing Practice and Health Policy Issues

Pamela Brown
  President and PhD, RN, Chief Executive Officer
  Blessing-Rieman College of Nursing

Janet Y. Harris MSN, RN, NEA-BC
  Chief Nurse Executive Officer and Interim Chief Executive Officer
  University of Mississippi Health Care

Joanne V. Hickey, PhD, RN, APRN, ACNP-BC, FAAN
  Professor Patricia L. Starck/PARTNERS Professorship in Nursing;
    Coordinator, Doctor of Nursing Practice Program
  University of Texas, School of Nursing

Kim W. Hoover, PhD, RN
  Dean and Professor
  University of Mississippi Medical Center School of Nursing

Pamela A. Kulbok, DNSc, RN, PHCNS-BC, FAAN
  Professor of Nursing and Public Health Sciences; Chair, Department of
    Family, Community, and Mental Health Systems; Coordinator of Public
    Health Nursing Leadership
  University of Virginia School of Nursing

Beth Martin, RN, MSN, CCNS, ACNP-BC, ACHPN
Nurse Practitioner
Hospice and Palliative Care, Charlotte Region

Brenda L. Lyon, PhD, RN, FAAN
Professor
Adult Health Department; Indiana School of Nursing

Jennifer Matthews, PhD, RN, A-CNS, CNE, FAAN
Professor, Clinical Nurse Specialist; Adult Health Certified Nurse Educator
Lead Nurse Planner, Continuing Education
Shenandoah University

Catherine E. Neuman, MSN, RN, NEA-BC
Nurse Consultant

Linda L. Olson, PhD, RN, NEA-BC
Director of Institute of Regulatory Excellence Fellowship Program;
National Council of State Boards of Nursing

Sharon J. Olsen, PhD, RN, AOCN
Assistant Professor
Johns Hopkins University, School of Nursing

Mary-Anne D. Ponti, RN, MSN, MBA, CNAA, FACHE
Chief Operating Officer and Chief Nurse Executive
Northern Michigan Regional Health System

Julie Stanik-Hutt, PhD, ACNP/GNP, CCNS, FAAN
Director, Master's Program Associate Professor and Coordinator, Adult-
Gerontology Acute Care, Nurse Practitioner Track
The Johns Hopkins University, School of Nursing

Margaret G. Williams PhD, RN, CNE
Professor, Blessing-Rieman College of Nursing

About the American Nurses Association

The American Nurses Association (ANA) is the only full-service professional organization representing the interests of the nation's 3.1 million registered nurses through its constituent/state nurses associations and its organizational affiliates. The ANA advances the nursing profession by fostering high standards of nursing practice, promoting the rights of nurses in the workplace, projecting a positive and realistic view of nursing, and by lobbying the Congress and regulatory agencies on health care issues affecting nurses and the public.

About Nursesbooks.org, The Publishing Program of ANA

Nursesbooks.org publishes books on ANA core issues and programs, including ethics, leadership, quality, specialty practice, advanced practice, and the profession's enduring legacy. Best known for the foundational documents of the profession on nursing ethics, scope and standards of practice, and social policy, Nursesbooks.org is the publisher for the professional, career-oriented nurse, reaching and serving nurse educators, administrators, managers, and researchers as well as staff nurses in the course of their professional development.

Introduction

The American Nurses Association (ANA) successfully champions professional nursing excellence (1) by defining the nursing profession's accountability to the public and the outcomes for which registered nurses are responsible and (2) by developing and implementing standards of practice and professional performance and a code of ethics. The goal of ANA is to develop and disseminate the cornerstone work of ANA as foundational for the profession. These cornerstones are *Nursing's Social Policy Statement: The Essence of the Profession* (ANA, 2010a), *Code of Ethics for Nurses with Interpretive Statements* (ANA, 2001), and *Nursing: Scope and Standards of Nursing Practice*, 2nd Edition (ANA, 2010b). Together, they comprehensively describe the competent level of practice for all registered nurses.

Nursing's Social Policy Statement (ANA, 2010a) describes the social contract between society and the profession of nursing and will be discussed in greater detail in chapter 1. The statement also defines nursing, describes the scope of practice and nursing roles and the regulation of nursing practice, and provides a good general reference for students and practicing nurses regarding the profession's responsibilities.

The current code of ethics for the profession, *Code of Ethics for Nurses with Interpretive Statements* (ANA, 2001), provides a reference for ethical decision-making and is the profession's expression of nursing's values, duties, and commitments to that public. The Code of Ethics for Nurses has nine ethical provisions, and they each delineate what nurses owe not only to others but also to themselves as members of a trusted profession. The Code of Ethics for Nurses was written as a living document for nurses, but the basic tenets found within each part of the code remain unchanged. Because of health care's continued evolution and complexity, another resource titled *Guide to the Code of Ethics for Nurses: Interpretation and Application* (Fowler, 2008) provides interpretation and examples of the application of the nine ethical provisions as they relate to today's practice.

The other foundational document is *Nursing: Scope and Standards of Practice*, 2nd Edition (ANA, 2010b). This important document describes the Standards of Practice and the Standards of Professional Performance, as well as the Scope of Nursing Practice. The delineation of that scope addresses the full range of practice activities that are common to all registered nurses. The six Standards of Practice are assessment, diagnosis, outcomes identification, planning, implementation, and evaluation. The ten Standards of Professional Performance are ethics, education, evidence-based practice and research, quality of practice, communication, leadership, collaboration, professional practice evaluation, resource utilization, and environmental health.

The ANA Congress on Nursing Practice and Economics (CNPE) has responsibility for the development and continued refinement of these foundational documents. The Committee on Nursing Practice Standards and Guidelines is given authority to function from the CNPE and has established a process for periodic review and revision of the scope and standards of practice.

Members of the Committee on Nursing Practice Standards and Guidelines are nursing leaders who are from the state nursing associations and who possess diverse experience with practice and special issues. The committee functions to identify standards issues that affect nursing practice, and it is responsible for managing the practice standards program for ANA. Committee members serve as first reviewers for the designation of new nursing specialties, and they review new or revised scopes and standards of practice from nursing specialty organizations. After reviewing, the committee makes a recommendation to the CNPE for recognition of a specialty, approval of scope statements, and acknowledgment of specialty standards. The committee uses a document, *Recognition of a Specialty, Approval of Scope Statements, and Acknowledgment of Nursing Practice Standards,* to guide its work. This document is available to specialty nursing organizations engaged in preparation of specialty scope and standards of practice.

Each chapter of this book and its accompanying presentation in PowerPoint format* have been written so each can be used on its own. In addition, each of the standards chapters is uniformly structured and provides the following:

- Underlying definitions, concepts, processes, and other information necessary for understanding the standard

- Applications of the standard in education, administration, quality improvement, and research

- One or more case studies and accompanying discussion topics

- References and resources

---

*This content is delivered online as part of product purchase: www.nursesbooks.org/EssentialGuidesPowerPoints

Whether used as educational or professional development course material or as a professional resource by practitioners, this book—the latest addition to ANA's important foundational documents—will serve as a guide to practitioners, educators, and administrators on how to use and apply Scope of Nursing Practice and the Standards of Practice and the Standards of Professional Performance in everyday practice at all levels of nursing.

—Kathleen M. White, PhD, RN, NEA-BC, FAAN

—Ann O'Sullivan, MSN, RN, NE-BC, CNE

References

American Nurses Association. (2001). *Code of Ethics for Nurses with interpretive statements*. Washington, DC: Nursesbooks.org.

American Nurses Association. (2010a). *Nursing's social policy statement: The essence of the profession*. Silver Spring, MD: Nursesbooks.org.

American Nurses Association. (2010b). *Nursing: Scope and standards of nursing practice, 2nd edition*. Silver Spring, MD: Nursesbooks.org.

Fowler, M. (Ed.). (2008). *Guide to the Code of Ethics for Nurses: Interpretation and application*. Silver Spring, MD: American Nurses Association.

CHAPTER 1

Nursing's Social Policy Statement

Catherine E. Neuman, MSN, RN, NEA-BC

Overview

Nursing is a part of the society from which it grew and continues to evolve. As a profession, nursing is valued both within and outside that society. From the time of Florence Nightingale's *Notes on Nursing: What It Is and What It Is Not* in 1859 and the work of Virginia Henderson in 1961, the nursing profession has been responsive to the needs of society. Continuing this tradition, in 1980 the American Nurses Association (ANA) published the first *Nursing: A Social Policy Statement* (ANA, 1980), which was updated in 1995 as *Nursing's Social Policy Statement*. In 2003, ANA published the second edition of *Nursing's Social Policy Statement*. Subsequently in 2010, ANA published *Nursing's Social Policy Statement: The Essence of the Profession* (ANA, 2010a), which articulates the ways in which contemporary nursing as a profession is valued within U.S. society and is uniquely accountable to that society. As with its predecessors, the current edition provides helpful information to nurses, other health professionals, legislators, regulators, members of funding bodies, and the public. This new guide presents a summary of each section, followed by a discussion of how each social policy statement applies to nursing practice.

Social Context of Nursing

Nursing continues to evolve, but it has always been an essential part of the society from which it grew. Nursing is responsible to society because its professional interests must be perceived as serving the interests of society. Professions, including nursing, are the property of society, not of the individual. What individuals acquire through training (education) is professional knowledge and skill, not a profession or even part ownership of one (Page, 1975, p. 7).

Nursing is dynamic rather than static and reflects the changing nature of society's needs. As health care continues to be of utmost importance in the United States and throughout the world, nursing provides a leadership role in guiding the public and political leaders in the following areas:

- *Organization, delivery, and financing quality health care*
  Quality health care is a human right for all (ANA, 2008). It is expected that healthcare professionals address the increasing costs of health care; the ongoing health disparities; and the continuing lack of safe, accessible, and available healthcare resources and services.

- *Provision for the public's health*
  This provision promotes the responsibility of nursing to supply basic self-help measures for all, and it enhances the use of health promotion, disease prevention, and environmental measures.

- *Expansion of nursing and healthcare knowledge and appropriate application of technology*
  Evidence-based practice, including the incorporation of research and evidence into nursing practice, promotes the application of knowledge and technology into healthcare outcomes.

- *Expansion of healthcare resources and health policy*
  Expanded facilities and workforce capacity for personal care and community services are required to accomplish this goal.

- *Definitive planning for health policy and regulation*
  Collaborative planning must be responsive to the needs of healthcare consumers and must provide resources for the health care of all members of society.

- *Duties under extreme conditions*
  Healthcare professionals provide care under extreme conditions, thereby weighing their obligation to provide care with their own health and that of their families during emergencies.

Social and political priorities for nursing include addressing the cost and quantity of healthcare services, along with having regulatory bodies provide various types of guidance. For example, both The Joint Commission and the Centers for

Medicare and Medicaid Services (CMS) set standards for expected quality of care. Others, such as the Agency for Healthcare Research and Quality (AHRQ) and the Institute for Healthcare Improvement (IHI), provide guidelines and protocols to attain quality and better outcomes.

Authority for nursing is based on a social responsibility, which derives from a complex social base and social contract. Nursing's social contract reflects the long-standing core values and ethics of the profession, which provide grounding for health care in society.

> *There is a social contract between society and the profession. Under its terms, society grants the profession's authority over functions vital to itself and permits them considerable autonomy in the conduct of their own affairs. In turn, the professions are expected to act responsibly, always mindful of the public trust. Self-regulation to assure quality and performance is at the heart of this relationship. It is the authentic hallmark of the mature profession. (Donabedian, 1976, p. 8)*

Today's contemporary society—as a result of apathy, depersonalization, disconnectedness, and growing globalization—sometimes encourages nursing to overlook this contract. Society validates the existence of the nursing profession through licensure, legal and legislative parameters, and public affirmation. This profession fulfills the need of society for qualified individuals who provide care according to a strong code of ethics to all in need, regardless of their social, cultural, or economic status.

The public has recognized nursing as one of the most-trusted professions. This trusted position imposes a responsibility to provide the very best health care, which requires well-educated, clinically astute nurses and a professional association composed of those nurses, which establishes a code of ethics, standards of care and practice, educational and practice requirements, and policies that govern the profession. The ANA, which is the professional organization for nurses, performs a critical function in articulating, maintaining, and strengthening the social contract that exists between nursing and society, thereby supporting the authority to practice nursing. Elements that undergird nursing's social contract with society include the following (ANA, 2010a, pp. 6–7):

- Humans manifest an essential unity of mind, body, and spirit.

- Human experience is contextually and culturally defined.

- Health and illness are human experiences. The presence of illness does not preclude health, nor does optimal health preclude illness.

- The relationship between the nurse and patient occurs within the context of the values and beliefs of the patient and nurse.

- Public policy and the healthcare delivery system influence the health and well-being of society and professional nursing.

- Individual responsibility and interprofessional involvement are essential.

The nursing profession focuses on establishing effective working relationships and collaborative efforts, which are essential to accomplishing its health-oriented mission. Many factors contribute to intensifying the importance of direct human interactions, communication, and professional collaboration: the complexity, size, and culture of the healthcare system and its transitional, dynamic state; an increase in public interest and involvement in health policy; and a national focus on health. Collaboration means true partnerships—partnerships that value expertise, power, and respect for all and partnerships that recognize and accept separate and combined spheres of activity and responsibility. To be successful in this arena, nursing needs to respond to diversity by recognizing, assessing, and adapting the nature of working relationships. Such relationships may be with individuals, with populations, with other health professionals, and with health workers, both within and between nurses and public representatives in all areas where nursing is practiced.

Definition of Nursing

Florence Nightingale (1859, p. 9) defined nursing as having charge of the personal health of somebody: "And what nursing has to do . . . is to put the patient in the best condition for nature to act upon him."

Later, Virginia Henderson (1960, p. 42) defined the purpose of nursing: "to assist the individual, sick or well, in the performance of those activities contributing to health or its recovery (or peaceful death) that he would perform unaided if he had the necessary strength, will, or knowledge, and to do this in such a way as to help him gain independence as rapidly as possible."

Nursing was defined in the original *Nursing: A Social Policy Statement* (ANA, 1980, p. 9) as "the diagnosis and treatment of human responses to actual or potential health problems." The current definition in the 2010 *Nursing's Social Policy Statement: The Essence of the Profession* remains unchanged from that in the 2004 edition:

> *Nursing is the protection, promotion, and optimization of health and abilities; prevention of illness and injury; alleviation of suffering through*

*the diagnosis and treatment of human response; and advocacy in the
care of individuals, families, communities, and populations. (ANA,
2010b, p. 10)*

This definition encompasses four essential characteristics of nursing: human
responses or phenomena, theory application, nursing actions or interventions,
and outcomes:

- *Human responses* are the responses of individuals to actual or potential
  health problems of concern to nurses, including any observable need,
  concern, condition, event, or fact of interest that may be the target of
  evidence-based nursing practice.

- *Theory application* is built on understanding theories of nursing and
  other disciplines as a basis for evidence-based nursing actions.

- *Nursing actions* are theoretically derived and evidence-based
  and require well-developed intellectual competencies. Their
  goal is to protect, promote, and optimize health; to prevent illness
  and injury; to alleviate suffering; and to advocate for all
  populations.

- *Outcomes of nursing actions* produce beneficial results in relation to
  identified human responses. Evaluation of those actions determines
  whether they have been effective. Findings from nursing research
  provide rigorous scientific evidence of beneficial outcomes of specific
  nursing actions.

Knowledge Base for Nursing Practice

Nursing is both a science and an art. Professional nursing practice requires
the nurse to have an understanding of nursing science, philosophy, and ethics; of biology and psychology; and of the social, physical, economic, organizational, and technological sciences. Nurses are expected to expand nursing's
knowledge base by using theories that are congruent with nursing values and
nursing practice.

Nurses are concerned with human experiences and responses across the
life span. They use theoretical and evidence-based knowledge of human
experiences and responses to collaborate with healthcare consumers and
others to assess, diagnose, identify outcomes, plan, implement, and evaluate care.

Regulation of Nursing Practice

Society grants authority over functions vital to the profession of nursing on the basis of the social contract between society and the profession, and society allows for considerable autonomy in the conduct of its own affairs. Like other professions, nursing is responsible for ensuring that its members act in the public interest while providing the unique service that society has entrusted to them. Processes that promote that end include professional, legal, and self-regulation.

PROFESSIONAL REGULATION

Professional regulation is the oversight, monitoring, and control of members on the basis of principles, guidelines, and rules deemed important by the profession. Professional regulation of nursing practice begins with the definition of professional nursing and the scope of professional nursing practice. The social contract for nursing has been made explicit through the work and collective expertise of the American Nurses Association, its constituent associations, and other nursing organizations. Those responsibilities include the following:

- Establishing and maintaining a professional code of ethics

- Determining standards of practice

- Fostering the development of nursing theory derived from nursing research

- Establishing nursing practice built on a base of best evidence

- Establishing the specifications for the educational requirements for entry into professional practice at basic and advanced levels

- Developing certification processes as measures of professional competence (ANA 2010a, p. 29)

LEGAL REGULATION

Legal regulation is the oversight, monitoring, and control of designated professionals on the basis of applicable statutes and regulations and accompanied by the interpretation of those laws. Nurses are legally accountable for both the actions taken in the course of their professional practice and those actions delegated to others who are assisting in the provision of nursing care. Accountability is accomplished through the legal regulatory mechanisms of licensure; the granting authority to practice, as through nurse practice acts;

and the criminal and civil laws. Thus, the legal contract between society and the nursing profession is defined by statute and associated rules and regulations. State nurse practice acts grant nurses the authority to practice and grant society the authority to sanction nurses who violate the norms of the profession or act in a manner that threatens the safety of the public. Statutory definitions of nursing should be compatible and should build on the profession's definition of its practice base.

SELF-REGULATION

Self-regulation requires personal accountability for the knowledge base for professional practice and is the individual's demonstrated personal control. As such, it is based on principles, guidelines, and rules. Nurses expect to develop and maintain current knowledge, skills, and abilities through formal academic programs and professional development programs. Certification in their area of practice is often pursued to demonstrate competence. Within their scope of practice, nurses exercise autonomy. Autonomy is defined as the capacity of a nurse to determine his or her own actions through independent choice within the full scope of nursing practice (Ballou, 1998). Nursing competency is an expected level of performance that integrates knowledge, skills, abilities, and judgment (ANA, 2008b). Competence is foundational to autonomy. Greater autonomy and freedom in nursing practice are based on broader authority that is rooted in advanced knowledge and competence in selected areas of nursing. Nurses regulate their own practice by participating in peer review and continuous performance improvement, both of which foster the refinement of knowledge, skills, and clinical decision-making processes at all levels and areas of professional nursing practice.

Use of the Social Policy Statement in Practice

Nursing's Social Policy Statement: The Essence of the Profession is essential for all nurses to understand nursing as it is defined, nursing as a profession, nursing process, nursing regulation, and advanced nursing practice. The definition of nursing, as cited earlier in this chapter, is used in legal, practice, education, and scope of practice documents. The essence of the profession of nursing—formalized and defined in the 2010 document—provides the basis for nursing practice. The nursing process has long been the critical thinking model for the profession and the basis for assessment, diagnosis, outcomes identification, planning, implementation, and evaluation. The profession has consciously reaffirmed the importance of the nursing process in the care of healthcare consumers.

The definition of nursing specialties, which forms the basis of recognition for those specialties, is also delineated herein. In fact, advanced nursing practice and advanced specialized nursing practice are defined and differentiated. This guide thus provides the basis for legal regulation and health policy for all nurses.

Members of the nursing faculty will find the content of the social policy statement useful in all levels of nursing education. Students will benefit from reviewing that statement as they learn about the evolution of their profession through its key attributes, the definition of nursing, the profession's description of the characteristics of a nursing specialty, and the delineation of its scope of practice and accompanying standards and competency statements. Such competency statements will provide them with assistance and understanding of the complexity of nursing practice. The social policy statement will also provide them with a clear delineation of the six social concerns in health care that undergird nursing's social contract with society. In addition, the social policy statement reaffirms the importance of collaboration within nursing and interprofessional teams.

The social policy statement may be used in professional development to reinforce the concepts of autonomy and competence and to address the importance of the scope of nursing practice, the nursing process, and the use of the standards of practice and professional performance in an everyday practice setting.

Nurse leaders and administrators will find the social policy statement very beneficial as a resource for strategic planning, vision and mission statements, and presentations about nurses and nursing. It is also valuable to members of legal and regulatory bodies to better understand how professional, self, and legal regulations complement each other.

Researchers may use the statement to provide a historical perspective of the definition of nursing. It also provides valuable insights related to the social context of nursing.

Conclusion

The social policy statement describes the pivotal nature and role of professional nursing in society and health care. Registered nurses focus their specialized knowledge, skills, and caring on improving the health status of the public and on ensuring safe, effective, quality care. The statement serves as a resource to assist nurses in conceptualizing the professional practice of nursing, and it provides direction to educators, administrators, and researchers within nursing. It also informs other health professionals, legislators, other regulators, funding bodies, and the public about nursing's responsibility, accountability, and contribution to health care. It assists in better understanding the foundation on which the nursing profession and registered nurses base their practice.

Discussion Topics

1. Describe the six social concerns in health care and nursing.

2. Describe the social contract between society and the profession of nursing.

3. On what is the authority of nursing based?

4. What is the definition of nursing?

5. List and discuss four essential characteristics of nursing.

6. Under the terms of the social contract between society and the profession of nursing, society grants authority over functions vital to the profession and permits considerable autonomy in the conduct of its own affairs. Professional nursing is accountable for ensuring that its members act in the public interest while providing the service society has entrusted to them. Discuss those processes.

7. In a clinical situation in your practice, identify specific ways that you can apply the social contract with healthcare consumers and the public.

References and Other Sources

American Nurses Association (ANA). (1980). *Nursing: A social policy statement*. Kansas City, MO: Author.

American Nurses Association (ANA). (2008a). *ANA's health system reform agenda*. Retrieved from http://www.nursingworld.org/ MainMenuCategories/HealthcareandPolicyIssues/HealthSystemReform/ Agenda.aspx

American Nurses Association. (2008b). *Professional role competence.*
http://www.nursingworld.org/MainMenuCategories/
ThePracticeofProfessionalNursing/NursingStandards/Professional-Role-
Competence.html

American Nurses Association (ANA). (2010a). *Nursing's social
policy statement: The essence of the profession.* Silver Spring,
MD: Nursesbooks.org.

American Nurses Association (ANA). (2010b). *Nursing: Scope and standards
of practice* (2nd ed.). Silver Spring, MD: Nursesbooks.org.

American Nurses Association (ANA). (2010c). *Recognition of a nursing
specialty, approval of a specialty nursing scope of practice statement, and
acknowledgment of specialty nursing standards of practice.* (Approved
by the Congress on Nursing Practice and Economics September 2010.)
Retrieved from http://www.nursingworld.org/MainMenuCategories/
ThePracticeofProfessionalNursing/NursingStandards/3-S-Booklet.aspx

Ballou, K. A. (1998). Concept analysis of autonomy. *Journal of Professional
Nursing, 14*(2), 102–110.

Donabedian, A. (1976). Foreword. In M. Phaneuf, *The nursing audit:
Self-regulation in nursing practice* (2nd ed., p. 8). New York:
Appleton-Century-Crofts.

Henderson, V. (1960). *Basic principles of nursing care.* London: International
Council of Nurses.

Nightingale, F. (1859). *Notes on nursing: What it is and what it is not*
(Preface, p. 75). London: Harrison and Sons. (Facsimile ed., 1946,
Philadelphia: J. B. Lippincott & Co.).

Page, B. B. (1975). Who owns the profession? *Hastings Center Report,
5*(5 October), 7–8.

CHAPTER 2

Scope of Nursing Practice

Ann O'Sullivan, MSN, RN, CNE, NE-BC

Overview of Scope of Nursing Practice

As discussed in chapter 1, the definition of nursing, according to the American Nurses Association (ANA, 2010a, p. 6), serves as the foundation for and is integral to understanding the details presented in *Nursing: Scope and Standards of Practice*, 2nd edition (ANA, 2010b).

> *A professional nursing organization has a responsibility to its members and to the public it serves to develop the scope and standards of its profession's practice. As the professional organization for all registered nurses, the American Nurses Association (ANA) has assumed the responsibility for developing the scope and standards [with broad input from the profession] that apply to the practice of all professional nurses and serve as a template for nursing specialty practice. (ANA, 2010b, p. 1)*

The scope of practice statement published by the ANA builds on that definition of nursing to succinctly and comprehensively describe the "who," "what," "where," "when," "why," and "how" of nursing practice. Each of those questions must be sufficiently answered to provide a complete picture of the dynamic and complex practice of nursing and its evolving boundaries and membership. The profession of nursing has one scope of practice that encompasses the full range of nursing practice. The depth and breadth in which individual registered nurses engage in the total scope of nursing practice depends on their education, experience, role, and the population served (ANA, 2010b, p. 2).

All nurses must understand what scope of practice means and must have the autonomy to practice to the full extent of their nursing license. The importance of scope of practice was identified as a key message in the Institute of Medicine's *Future of Nursing* report (IOM, 2011; p. 5): "Regulatory barriers are particularly problematic. Regulations defining scope-of-practice limitations vary widely by state. As a result, what advanced practice registered nurses are able to do once they graduate varies widely for reasons that are related not to their ability, education or training, or safety concerns, but to the political decisions of the state in which they work." The report makes a bold recommendation to "Remove scope-of-practice barriers. Advanced practice registered nurses should be able to practice to the full extent of their education and training. Specific actions are suggested for how to accomplish this recommendation" (IOM, 2011; p. 271). Although this recommendation primarily addresses the scope of practice for nurse practitioners, *all* nurses should practice to the full extent of their scope of practice.

Nursing Process

The nursing process, a key framework for nursing, is the method for carrying out the scope of practice by the professional nurse. It relies heavily on feedback loops among the components of the process: assessment (Standard 1), diagnosis (Standard 2), outcomes identification (Standard 3), planning (Standard 4), implementation (Standard 5), and evaluation (Standard 6), as illustrated in Figure 2.1. The nursing process is used in both clinical and nonclinical settings and practice roles.

In the clinical setting, the nurse on a surgical unit uses the nursing process feedback loop in caring for a patient who is in pain after surgery. After providing pain treatment, the nurse reassesses the patient's pain to determine whether the treatment has relieved the pain. If the pain is not relieved or controlled, the nurse continues to assess, to develop outcomes, and to plan and implement new measures to control the pain. The nurse continues to reassess and evaluate those measures with the patient until the patient's pain is under control.

In nursing education, the instructor uses several assessment tools and processes to identify a student's knowledge, skills, and abilities in a specific area of nursing practice. The instructor identifies outcomes according to the specific content and the student's level of experience and education. Next, the instructor develops and implements plans to meet identified outcomes and then reassesses periodically through testing, clinical observation, and discussions with the student. Drawing on further assessments, plans, and implementation, the instructor may revise strategies. Evaluation is ongoing.

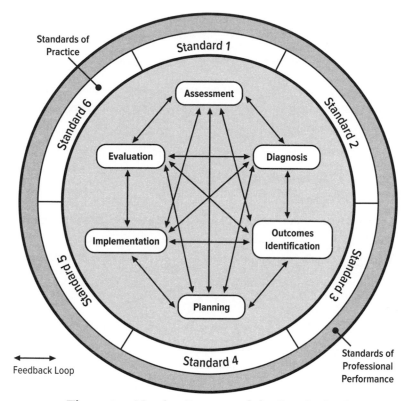

Figure 2.1. Nursing Process and the Standards of
Professional Nursing Practice (ANA, 2010b, p. 3)

Further examples of how each step of the nursing process and the corresponding Standard of Practice is used in nursing practice are included in each of the chapters dealing with Standards 1–6.

Characteristics of Nursing Practice

ANA's discussion of the Scope of Nursing Practice identifies tenets of professional nursing practice (ANA, 2010b, pp. 4–5). A tenet is an axiomatic principle or belief generally held as true, usually in the context of an organization, profession, or other such group. The five tenets of professional nursing practice are as follows:

1. Nursing practice is individualized.

2. Nurses coordinate care by establishing partnerships.

3. Caring is central to the practice of the registered nurse.

4. Registered nurses use the nursing process to plan and provide individualized care to their healthcare consumers.

5. A strong link exists between the professional work environment and the registered nurse's ability to provide quality health care and achieve optimal outcomes.

Model of Professional Nursing Practice Regulation

In 2006, the Model of Professional Nursing Practice Regulation (see figure 2.2) emerged from ANA work and informed the regulatory discussions addressing nursing, specialty nursing, and advanced practice registered nursing

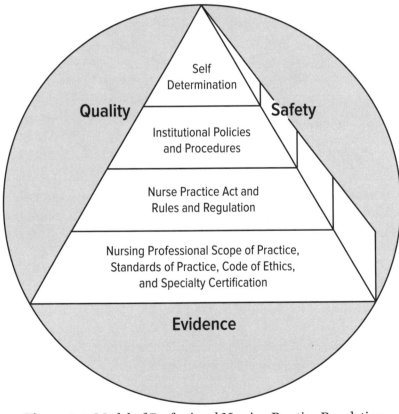

Figure 2.2. Model of Professional Nursing Practice Regulation (Styles, Schumann, Bickford, & White, 2008, p. 21)

practice. The lowest level in the model represents the responsibility of the professional and specialty nursing organizations to their members and the public to define the scope and standards of practice for nursing. The next level up the pyramid represents the regulation provided by the nurse practice act, rules, and regulations in the pertinent licensing jurisdictions. Institutional policies and procedures provide further directions for the registered nurse and the advanced practice registered nurse in the regulation of nursing practice. Note the highest level is that of self-determination, which is made by individual nurses about their competency and scope of practice after they consider all the other levels of input about professional nursing practice regulation.

Nurse Practice Acts

Many state nurses associations and other professional nursing groups have helped revise state nurse practice acts to reflect ANA's Scope and Standards of Nursing, which has been determined by the profession. This approach requires ongoing education and lobbying of state legislators, boards of nursing, state regulatory agencies, and other providers of health care. Revisions that make state laws and the profession's definition of the scope of practice congruent are particularly helpful for the public and the profession.

For example, the scope of practice statement in the Illinois Nurse Practice Act (IDFPR 2007) is congruent with the ANA definition because of the lobbying efforts of the nurses in Illinois and is defined in the following paraphrase:

1. The comprehensive nursing assessment of the health status of patients that addresses changes to patient conditions.

2. The development of a plan of nursing care to be integrated within the patient-centered healthcare plan that establishes nursing diagnoses and the setting of goals to meet identified healthcare needs, to determine nursing interventions, and to implement nursing care through the execution of nursing strategies and regimens ordered or prescribed by authorized healthcare professionals.

3. The administration of medication or delegation of medication administration to licensed practical nurses.

4. The delegation of nursing interventions to implement the plan of care.

5. The provision for the maintenance of safe and effective nursing care rendered directly or through delegation.

6. The act of advocating for patients.

7. The evaluation of responses to interventions and the effectiveness of the plan of care.

8. The act of communicating and collaborating with other healthcare professionals.

9. The procurement and application of new knowledge and technologies.

10. The provision of health education and counseling.

11. The participation in development of policies, procedures, and systems to support patient safety.

Institutional Policies and Procedures

Nurses must be involved in developing institutional policies and procedures that are up to date according to evidence, are reviewed regularly, and are easily accessible to all. Institutions must effectively communicate policies in a timely manner with the nursing staff and must share with new staff members during orientation. Healthy work environments are essential to nursing practice, both for nurses and for healthcare consumers. Institutional policies and procedures affect the context of these work environments. The following four approaches to designing such work environments address the critical issues of this topic.

AACN SIX STANDARDS

In 2001, the American Association of Critical-Care Nurses (AACN, 2005) developed six standards that can be a valuable resource to developing policies that establish and sustain healthy work environments, which will, in turn, support and foster excellence in patient care and be applied to all areas of nursing practice. The six standards focus on (1) skilled communication by nurses, (2) interprofessional collaboration, (3) effective decision-making, (4) appropriate staffing, (5) meaningful recognition, and (6) authentic leadership.

MAGNET RECOGNITION PROGRAM®

A second approach, the Magnet Recognition Program®, addresses the professional work environment, thereby requiring that Magnet-designated facilities adhere to five model components (ANCC, 2008). Those facilities use resources to organize and develop institutional policies and procedures, and they promote transformational leadership; structural empowerment; exemplary professional practice; new knowledge, innovation, and improvements; and empirical quality results.

14 FORCES OF MAGNETISM

A third approach, the Magnet program and its 14 Forces of Magnetism, can be applied to nursing education programs that improve the work environment for the faculty and staff members and the learning environment for students. These new Magnet Model Components include the 14 Forces of Magnetism, include language from the standards throughout, and require organizations that are seeking Magnet Recognition to use the standards to build their programs of nursing excellence. The 14 Forces of Magnetism (Drenkard, Wolf, & Morgan, 2011, pp. 26, 29) are as follows: nursing leadership and management style; professional development; image of nursing; organizational structure; personnel policies and programs; community; professional models of care; autonomy; interdisciplinary relations; consultation and resources; nurses as teachers; quality of care: ethics, patient safety, and quality infrastructure; quality improvement; and quality of care: research and evidence-based practice.

CLINICAL PRACTICE MODEL

And finally, the Clinical Practice Model (CPM) (Wesorick & Hanson, 2000) describes four characteristics of a healthy culture: shared purpose, meaningful conversation, healthy relationships, and supportive infrastructures. Without shared purpose, nurses lose the passion and purpose of the work. Without meaningful conversation, nurses lose the value of the collective wisdom of patients and colleagues. Without healthy relationships, people fail to connect at the human level, and cultures become dehumanized. Without system supports, people lose sight of what matters most and get caught up in the busyness all around. The CPM developed the Partnership Culture Model, which represents both the infrastructure and staff engagement environment necessary to deliver both the professional care in a transformed healthcare world and the culture of partnership in an organization and community. This partnership model is an example of shared governance where institutional policies and procedures can be developed by the interprofessional team.

Self-Determination

The Model of Professional Nursing Practice Regulation (see Figure 2.1 on p. 13) is an important aspect of the nurse's decision-making process regarding scope of practice in patient care. In every situation, the nurse must first consider the professional requirements and guidance as identified in ANA's Scope and Standards of Practice and in the nine provisions of the Code of Ethics for Nurses. The state nurse practice acts are developed to protect the public and should be derived from the professional scope and standards. Registered nurses and the organizations in which they are employed must be aware of and use professional standards and state laws and regulation to develop institutional policies and procedures.

After considering the professional standards of practice, the state nurse practice act and regulations, and the institutional policies and procedures for practice, nurses should consider the specific situation and clinical context, including their own education and experience; the staffing mix; the acuity of the healthcare consumer; the physical environment; and the availability of support systems, other providers, and emergency teams before they make a practice decision. Such an approach reflects self-determination.

Wesorick and Hanson's CPM (2000) describes nursing's unique professional services and could be useful as a model for nurses to determine what is in their scope of practice in particular situations:

1. Services that enhance the health of a person and require a physician's order. These delegated services are provided because the patient needs them (not simply because the physician orders them) and because the services require nursing knowledge and critical thinking.

2. Services that enhance the health of a person by assessing, monitoring, detecting, and preventing physiological complications associated with a medical diagnosis or treatment plan. These interdependent services are not driven by tasks, but, rather, are driven by making judgments and decisions, and they require nursing knowledge of the signs and symptoms of potential problems and prevention of complications.

3. Services that enhance health by assessing, monitoring, detecting, diagnosing, and treating human responses using nursing diagnosis. These independent services address the patients' wholeness and the body, mind, and spirit connection. The services require nursing knowledge to help the patient and family through their response to the diagnosis.

The CPM is a particularly helpful model that uses specific examples for describing the "what" of any particular scope of practice. Although other healthcare professionals also carry out the first two functions, the nursing profession has primary responsibility to healthcare consumers for the third function. For example, before delegating to another care provider, the nurse first considers the ANA Standards of Nursing Practice and the delegation competency in the

Resource Utilization standard of practice and Code of Ethics for Nurses provisions. Next, the nurse must know what the state law and rules and regulations for delegation allow in the state where he or she is practicing. Institutional policies will further direct how and what can be delegated to another care provider. And finally, the education, experience, and competence of the delegatee and the delegating nurse, plus the needs of the individual patient, will determine what is delegated to another person. All of these decision points are based on evidence and on working together to ensure safe and quality patient care.

Conclusion

The ANA Scope of Nursing Practice describes the who, what, where, when, why, and how of nursing practice. The profession has one scope of practice as described in the definition of nursing. The nursing process is the method the nurse uses for carrying out the scope of practice. Nurses use the Model of Professional Nursing Practice Regulation, starting with the Scope of Nursing Practice, state laws, institutional policies, and their self-determination to make decisions in their professional role. All nurses in all roles and settings must understand the scope of practice and must have the autonomy to practice to the full extent of their license.

Exercises for Application

1. Exercise for nursing students early in the semester:

For each of the following areas of the ANA Scope of Nursing Practice.

a. Identify what activities you observed your nurse do for four of her or his assigned patients.

b. Analyze what else could have been done for each patient in each area.

   i. Services that enhance the health of a person and require a physician's order.

   ii. Services that enhance the health of a person by assessing, monitoring, detecting, and preventing physiological complications associated with a medical diagnosis or treatment plan.

   iii. Services that enhance health by assessing, monitoring, detecting, diagnosing, and treating human responses using nursing diagnosis.

Personal evaluation:

    a. As a result of this critical thinking activity, I have learned . . .

    b. This activity gave me insights into the Scope of Nursing Practice because . . .

    c. This activity shows that I have more to learn about . . .

2. Exercise for upper-level nursing students:

For each of the following areas of the Nursing Scope of Practice,

    a. Identify nursing care you provided for your patients.

    b. Analyze what else you could have done for each patient in each area.

        i.   Services that enhance the health of a person and require a physician's order

        ii. Services that enhance the health of a person by assessing, monitoring, detecting, and preventing physiological complications associated with a medical diagnosis or treatment plan

        iii. Services that enhance health by assessing, monitoring, detecting, diagnosing, and treating human responses using nursing diagnosis

Personal Evaluation:

    a. As a result of this critical thinking activity, I have learned . . .

    b. This activity gave me insights into the Scope of Nursing Practice because . . .

    c. This activity shows that I have more to learn about . . .

3. Exercises for Nursing Regulation Pyramid Model:

First, analyze two clinical nursing actions (e.g., assessment, intervention, evaluation) you took today in caring for your patients according to the *Model of Professional Nursing Practice Regulation:*

    a. What is the standard according to the ANA Scope and Standards of Practice?

    b. What is the standard according to the nurse practice act in your state?

    c. What is the standard according to the institution's policy and procedure?

d. What and why did you choose the specific action you undertook?

e. How did this action enhance the quality and safety of patient care?

Then, analyze two nursing leadership or professional actions (e.g., delegation, communication, collaboration) you took today in caring for your patients according to the *Model of Professional Nursing Practice Regulation:*

a. What is the standard according to the ANA Scope and Standards of Practice?

b. What is the standard according to the nurse practice act in your state?

c. What is the standard according to the institution's policy and procedure?

d. What and why did you choose the specific action you undertook?

e. How did this action enhance the quality and safety of patient care?

Debbie Smith, RN, has floated to the emergency department to help out on the shift. She is assisting a nurse in caring for a trauma patient who has a respiratory arrest. The physician directs her to intubate the patient.

a. Is this intervention within her scope of practice?

b. How would she go about deciding whether to carry out this order?

References and Other Sources

American Association of Critical-Care Nurses (AACN). (2005). *AACN standards for establishing and maintaining healthy work environments.* Mission Viejo, CA: AACN. Retrieved from http://www.aacn.org/WD/HWE/Docs/HWEStandards.pdf

American Nurses Association (ANA). (2010a). *Nursing's social policy statement: The essence of the profession.* Silver Spring, MD: Nursesbooks.org

American Nurses Association (ANA). (2010b). *Nursing: Scope and standards of practice* (2nd ed.). Silver Spring, MD: Nursesbooks.org.

American Nurses Credentialing Center (ANCC). (2008). *A new model for ANCC's Magnet Recognition Program.* Silver Spring, MD: Author.

Drenkard, K., Wolf G., & Morgan, S. (Eds.) (2011). *Magnet®: The next generation—Nurses making the difference*. Silver Spring, MD: American Nurses Credentialing Center, Magnet Recognition Program®.

Gallagher-Lepak, S., & Kubsch, S. (2009). Transpersonal caring: A nursing practice guideline. *Holistic Nursing Practice, 23*, 171–182.

Hagerty, B. M. K., Lynch-Sauer, K., Patusky, K. L., & Bouwseman, M. (1993). An emerging theory of human relatedness. *Image, 25*, 291–296.

Illinois Department of Financial and Professional Regulation (IDFPR). (2007). Illinois Nurse Practice Act. 225ILCS 65 (October 5, 2007). Chicago, IL: Author. Retrieved from http://www.idfpr.com/profs/info/Nursing.asp

Institute of Medicine (IOM). (2011). *The future of nursing: Leading change, advancing health*. Washington, DC: Author. Retrieved from http://www.nap.edu/catalog/12956.html

Koloroutis, M. (2004). *Relationship-based care: A model for transforming practice*. Minneapolis, MN: Creative Health Care Management.

Styles, M. M., Schumann, M. J., Bickford, C. J., & White, K. M. (2008). *Specialization and credentialing in nursing revisited: Understanding the issues, advancing the profession*. Silver Spring, MD: Nursesbooks.org.

Swanson, K. (1993). Nursing as informed caring for the well-being of others. *Journal of Nursing Scholarship, 25*(4), 352–357.

Watson, J. (1999). *Postmodern nursing and beyond*. Edinburgh: Churchill Livingstone.

Watson, J. (2008). *Nursing: The philosophy and science of caring*. Boulder, CO: University Press of Colorado.

Wesorick, B., & Hanson, D. (2000). *Clinical practice guidelines*. Grand Rapids, MI: Practice Field Publishing.

CHAPTER 3
Standards of Nursing Practice

Kathleen M. White, PhD, RN, NEA-BC, FAAN

Nursing as a Profession

The classic definition of a professional association is "an organization of practitioners who judge one another as professionally competent and who have banded together to perform social functions which they cannot perform in their separate capacity as individuals" (Merton, 1958). As the professional association representing all registered nurses, the American Nurses Association (ANA) has the responsibility to describe the scope and standards of practice for all registered nurses.

In writing about nursing as a profession, Richard Hall (1968) described a professional model with five indicators of an individual's attitude toward professionalism. The attitudinal attributes are (1) use of a professional organization as the major source of ideas and judgments for the professional, (2) belief that the profession was created to serve the public, (3) belief that the profession must be self-regulating, (4) belief in a sense of calling to the work of the profession, and (5) belief in the importance of autonomy in decision-making about work. These attributes remain relevant to the present-day discussion about the important role that the professional organization plays in setting standards for the practice of that profession (standards of practice). His work also emphasizes the need for each profession to develop its own method of measuring professionalism (standards of professional performance).

Cyril Houle (1980) studied the functions that professions perform in relation to society and suggested that three groups of characteristics reflect the professionalization of an occupation: conceptual, performance, and collective identity. An important characteristic of a profession is the ability to develop a credentialing system and to certify competence. The conceptual characteristic of a profession is that a profession must be able to state and define its mission and foundations of practice. There are four characteristics of performance: mastery of theoretical knowledge, capacity to solve problems, use of practical knowledge, and self-enhancement. Finally, Houle defined nine characteristics within the collective identity: formal training, credentialing, subculture norms and values, legal reinforcement, public acceptance, ethical practice, penalties, relations to other vocations, and relations to users of the service.

The ANA defines and disseminates the responsibilities associated with the functions of a profession through three foundational publications—*Nursing's Social Policy Statement: The Essence of the Profession* (ANA, 2010a); *Code of Ethics for Nurses with Interpretive Statements* (ANA, 2001); and *Nursing: Scope and Standards of Practice*, 2nd Edition (ANA, 2010b). These publications define the accountability and autonomy that nursing has by virtue of its status as a profession. Nurses are accountable for their knowledge; skills; and behavior to self, to institution, to regulatory and legal entities, to the profession, to the healthcare consumer, and to society. They have autonomy to act independently and to make appropriate decisions as they relate to control over their own practice. This accountability and autonomy for practice are governed by nursing's scope and standards of practice.

Standards of Professional Nursing Practice

Standards are authoritative statements by which the nursing profession describes the responsibilities for which its practitioners are accountable. Standards reflect the values and priorities of the profession and provide both a direction for professional nursing practice and a framework for the evaluation of this practice. They also define the nursing profession's accountability to the public and the outcomes for which registered nurses are responsible (ANA, 2010b). Standards are important because they outline what is expected of a professional. The set of nursing standards published by ANA are formally designated as the Standards of Professional Nursing Practice, which contain the Standards of Practice and the Standards of Professional Performance. The competencies that accompany each standard may be evidence of compliance with the corresponding standard. This list of competency statements is not exhaustive for a given standard. Whether a particular standard or competency applies will depend on the circumstances.

The Standards of Practice "describe[s] a competent level of nursing care, as demonstrated by the critical thinking model known as the nursing process, which includes the components of assessment, diagnosis, outcomes identification, planning, implementation, and evaluation," and represents the problem-solving process that the registered nurse follows in daily interactions with patients, groups, communities, and systems. These standards "encompass significant actions taken by registered nurses and form the foundation of the nurse's decision-making." (ANA, 2010b, p. 9)

The Standards of Professional Performance "describe[s] a competent level of behavior in the professional role, including activities related to ethics, education, evidence-based practice and research, quality of practice, communication, leadership, collaboration, professional practice evaluation, resource utilization, and environmental health" (ANA, 2010b, p. 10). The Standards of Professional Performance describes how the registered nurse follows the Standards of Practice, completes the nursing process, and deals with other nursing practice issues as they arise in his or her career. "Registered nurses are accountable for their professional actions to themselves, their patients, their peers, and ultimately to society" (ANA, 2010b, p. 11).

Competence in nursing practice is an essential aspect of understanding and advancing the profession. Since the publication of the 2004 edition of *Nursing: Scope and Standards of Practice*, this topic has become even more prominent. A key portion of the 2010 scope of practice statement (ANA, 2010b, pp. 12–13) addresses this topic. Also, each of the standards is accompanied by a list of competency statements, which are key indicators—but not the only indicators—of competent practice for that standard.

ANA's 2008 position statement, *Professional Role Competence* (which is included as an appendix in the 2010 edition), articulates the importance of professional role competence in nursing:

> *The public has a right to expect registered nurses to demonstrate professional competence throughout their careers. ANA believes the registered nurse is individually responsible and accountable for maintaining professional competence. The ANA further believes that it is the nursing profession's responsibility to shape and guide any process for [ensuring] nurse competence. Regulatory agencies define minimal standards for regulation of practice to protect the public. The employer is responsible*

and accountable to provide an environment conducive to competent practice. Assurance of competence is the shared responsibility of the profession, individual nurses, professional organizations, credentialing and certification entities, regulatory agencies, employers, and other key stakeholders (ANA, 2008).

An individual who demonstrates competence is performing successfully at an expected level. A competency is an expected and measurable level of nursing performance that integrates knowledge, skills, abilities, and judgment, all of which are based on scientific knowledge and expectations for nursing practice (ANA, 2010b, p. 64). Formal, informal, and reflective learning experiences foster development of the requisite knowledge, skills, abilities, and judgment necessary for safe, high-quality nursing practice. Competence in nursing practice must be evaluated by the individual nurse (self-assessment); nurse peers; and nurses in the roles of supervisor, coach, mentor, or preceptor. In addition, other aspects of nursing performance may be evaluated by professional colleagues and by patients or clients.

The list of competency statements that accompany each standard may be evidence of compliance with the corresponding standard, but each list is not exhaustive. However, the selection of competency statements for each standard considered as a whole constitutes a minimum set of competencies applicable across all practice settings for all registered nurses. In addition, each standard except for one (the professional communication standard) also lists competencies unique to advanced practice by graduate-level prepared nurses and advanced practice registered nurses.

Application of the Standards to Nursing Practice

Nursing: Scope and Standards of Practice, 2nd Edition (ANA, 2010b), serves as the basis for many activities for nursing practice, including the development of nursing educational programs; role and specialty certification; policies, procedures, and protocols; position descriptions and performance appraisals; quality improvement activities; specialty nursing scope and standards of practice; legal and regulatory activities; and development and evaluation of nursing service delivery systems and organizational structures. Some applications of the 16 standards in nursing education, leadership and administration, performance and quality improvement, and research are discussed on the following pages. More specific insights into applications of each standard are provided in the 16 standards chapters that follow.

Education

In nursing education, the standards of practice and professional performance are used to guide curriculum development. Both the National League for Nursing Accrediting Commission and the Commission on Collegiate Nursing Education require use of national nursing standards for curriculum design and evaluation. The standards of practice and professional performance are one set of standards that can be used for curriculum design and evaluation. Examples of the use of the standards at each level of nursing education will be discussed.

Beginning-level nursing students should be introduced to the concept of standards of practice and the role of the ANA as the professional organization that is for nursing and that develops the standards. Examples of using the concept for these beginning students would be to develop class norms from the standards or to introduce the students to upper-level clinical tools and to how the standards (and the code of ethics) that were used in developing the tools.

As a follow-up, students should have a more in-depth discussion of the development and use of standards, of how the standards flow from the definition of nursing (ANA, 2010a, p. 10), and of how the standards relate to the scope of practice and the code of ethics. Development of clinical case studies for discussion in clinical conferences should include real-time use of standards in clinical experiences in long-term and acute care for the beginning-level interactions with patients. For example, beginning clinical experiences include performing a patient assessment.

Discussion of one or more of the competencies in Standard 1 Assessment should be included in the clinical conference. Begin with "[p]rioritizes data collection based on the healthcare consumer's immediate condition, or the anticipated needs of the healthcare consumer or situation" (ANA, 2010b, p. 32). For beginning students, discussion of the standard and this competency would center on how the student approaches the assessment (or has to stop and give the patient time to rest) on the basis of the patient's level of acuity and complexity. As the students begin their clinical experiences for the first time, they should see how the evaluation of their clinical performance is based on standards and is reflected in the development and use of the clinical evaluation tools.

Upper-level nursing students' experiences should begin with a discussion of the application of the scope of practice, standards, and code of ethics in the major practice areas included in all nursing education programs, such as obstetrics, pediatrics, medical–surgical, and psychiatric–mental health nursing. The standards of practice and any applicable specialty standards are also very useful in other practice areas, such as critical care, emergency department, and community health experiences.

Application of the standards in master's and doctoral-level education involve the use of the "Additional Competencies for the Graduate-Level Specialty Nurse or the Advanced Practice Registered Nurse" for each standard. Again for those students, the clinical evaluation tools should include the additional competencies and should be used to guide design and evaluation of the curriculum. For example, the students should be required to obtain and review the standards of practice and professional performance and their specialty practice standards. Classroom or clinical conference discussions should challenge such students to discuss how they meet the competencies for the registered nurse and to identify experiences for developing competency at the higher level and for evaluating the standards and competencies for their practice.

Administration

The Standards of Practice and Professional Performance have many uses in the administration of a nursing service organization, large or small. The Standards of Practice serve as the framework for an organization to develop its own standards of practice and professional performance. Those organizational standards guide the approach to nursing care within an organization and hold the individual nurse to professional, legal, and ethical obligations for practice. The standards provide an important framework for organizing and performing the work of nursing and for measuring the quality of that work. The standards also require that nurses assume accountability and responsibility for their own practices.

The standards should be used to guide the development of job descriptions, evaluation tools, and the orientation programs for the organization. A human resource program that uses the standards provides documents that flow from one another and that make sense to the employee and the manager. To begin, the standards should be used to describe the overall accountable categories in the job descriptions, and the competencies should provide the detail to measure the employee's success. Flowing from the job descriptions, the evaluation tools should have the same accountable categories (standards) and competencies for evaluation.

For example, Standard 11 Communication states, "The registered nurse communicates effectively in a variety of formats in all areas of practice" (ANA, 2010b, p. 54). The organization would develop an evaluation tool that includes a standard of care for all nurses about communication, and it could use the competency statements as printed in *Nursing: Scope and Standards of Practice*, 2nd Edition (ANA, 2010b). Or the organization could use the competency statements as a framework to develop its own statements of accountability such as the following:

The registered nurse

1. Demonstrates respect and mutual valuing toward other staff members and peers.

2. Creates positive interpersonal work environment.

3. Maintains confidentiality in communication with patients, family members, other health professionals, and staff members.

4. Conveys information to other team members to effectively manage patient care needs.

Finally, the organization's orientation program should be designed around those job descriptions and evaluation tools to provide the appropriate education and direction to new employees about organizational expectations and about job accountability and responsibilities.

The Magnet Recognition Program®, developed by the American Nurses Credentialing Center, recognizes healthcare organizations that provide and disseminate successful innovative nursing practices and that espouse nursing excellence (ANCC, 2012). A Magnet environment achieves quality indicators and nursing practice standards outlined in the *ANA Nursing Administration: Scope and Standards of Practice*, 3rd Edition (ANA, 2009) and other foundational documents. (The *ANA Nursing Administration: Scope and Standards of Practice*, 3rd Edition, is obviously based on *Nursing: Scope and Standards of Practice*, 2nd Edition [ANA, 2010b].)

Performance and Quality Improvement

The Standards of Professional Nursing Practice have an important role in performance and quality improvement efforts in healthcare organizations. The standards should establish the level of practice that forms the basis of the program and should be used to define, monitor, and measure patient outcomes. Nurses' knowledge of and accountability and responsibility for the Standards of Practice and Professional Performance also empower nurses to use their clinical knowledge and expertise to question practice and to lead practice improvements.

For example, Standard 6 Evaluation includes a competency to "[conduct] a systematic, ongoing, and criterion-based evaluation of the outcomes in relation to structures and processes prescribed by the plan of care and indicated timeline" (ANA, 2010b, p. 45); Standard 10 Quality of Practice includes a competency to "[participate] in quality improvement" (ANA, 2010b, p. 52). Those competencies directly relate to the work of performance improvement and hold the registered nurse accountable for monitoring and evaluating patient outcomes for improvement. Additionally, the standards also promote interprofessional practice and collaboration, which are a foundation to performance improvement efforts.

Research

Throughout the standards of practice, statements of accountability are included for nurses to develop, implement, and evaluate evidence-based nursing practice, research, and standards of care. To facilitate this process successfully, nurses are responsible and held accountable to maintain their nursing knowledge. Maintaining current knowledge includes the responsibility to develop, promote, and evaluate nursing knowledge and other healthcare research as they affect nursing practice.

Key Legal and Practical Implications of Standards

Many states have used the Standards of Practice and Standards of Professional Performance directly or in part to guide the development of their own state nurse practice act legislation or regulation, such as California, Delaware, District of Columbia, Florida, Hawaii, Illinois, Kansas, Kentucky, Louisiana, Maryland, Minnesota, Mississippi, Nevada, New Jersey, New Mexico, and Oklahoma. The state boards of nursing often defer to the professional standards when interpretation of practice is required. For example, ANA's Standards of Practice and Professional Performance or any nursing specialty standards that are based on the ANA standards will be used by the boards to accomplish the following:

- Develop the scope of practice statements for licensure.

- Expand the scope statements for advanced practice nurses.

- Make decisions about emerging new practices and procedures.

- Define new categories of licensure, recognition, or certification.

- Determine the appropriateness and level of discipline.

- Define state accreditation of nursing educational programs.

The Standards of Practice and Professional Performance are often used in state board of nursing actions and in nursing negligence and malpractice actions. When the standards are used in negligence and malpractice cases, they establish the standard of care, and legal authorities apply the standards to definitions that are used to decide negligence and malpractice, such as the following:

1. *Standard of care*—Defines what should or should not be done for a patient and is the level of care for which a nurse is held accountable.

2. *Duty*—Defines the relationship between the nurse and patient requiring the nurse to deliver care.

3. *Causation*—Is an act or omission that causes harm.

The standard of care that the nurse is accountable for is whether a "reasonably prudent nurse" would render the same care in the same or similar circumstance. A reasonable and prudent nurse is usually defined as a similarly educated and experienced nurse who has average intelligence, judgment, foresight, and skill and who would have responded to the same situation, case, facts, or emergency in the same or similar manner. Any nurse who does not meet the standard of care may be found negligent. Most legal actions involving a nurse occur because the nurse breached the standard of care.

Nursing Specialty Practice

In the late 1990s, the ANA partnered with other nursing organizations to establish a formal process for recognizing specialty areas of nursing practice. This process includes the criteria for approving the specialty itself, the scope statement, and the acknowledgment of standards of practice for that specialty. Three levels of ANA review are in this process. Because of the significant changes in the evolving nursing and healthcare environments, ANA's approval of specialty nursing scope statements and acknowledgment of specialty standards of practice remain valid for five years, starting from the publication date of the documents. ANA's Scope and Standards of Practice serve as a resource template for specialty nursing organizations when defining their practice domain. Often, specialty nursing organizations elect to clarify the uniqueness of their specialty nursing practice by publishing a specialty nursing scope and standards document. The nursing specialty credentialing organizations rely on the scope and standards when developing certification examinations and other components of the credentialing program.

ANA Recognition of Specialty

The following characteristics must be met for ANA recognition of a nursing specialty. A nursing specialty (ANA, 2010c) does the following:

- Defines itself as nursing.

- Adheres to the overall licensure requirements of the profession.

- Subscribes to the overall purposes and functions of nursing.

- Is clearly defined.

- Can identify a need and demand for itself.

- Has a well-derived knowledge base that is particular to the practice of that nursing specialty.

- Is concerned with phenomena of the discipline of nursing.

- Defines competencies for that area of specialty nursing practice.

- Has existing mechanisms for supporting, reviewing, and disseminating research to support its knowledge base.

- Has defined educational criteria for specialty preparation or a graduate degree.

- Has continuing education programs or continuing competence mechanisms for nurses in the specialty.

- Is organized and represented by a national or international specialty association or branch of a parent organization.

- Is practiced nationally or internationally.

- Includes a substantial number of registered nurses who devote most of their practice to the specialty.

Once those criteria are satisfied and the nursing specialty is recognized, *Nursing: Scope and Standards of Practice*, 2nd Edition (ANA, 2010b), serves as a template for the nursing specialty organization to define and describe the scope and standards of practice for the complexities of practice within the specialty.

Conclusion

Standards play a very important role in the everyday life of a professional. Society holds professionals accountable for their behavior and actions. Standards set forth what a profession expects of members; standards provide the overall framework for measuring the competency of the professional; and, for nursing, standards guide the nursing practice. The practice of nursing (general and specialty, basic and advanced) is dynamic and complex in today's healthcare environment. Practicing nurses must be aware of all standards of practice and professional performance and of the accountability and responsibility they have to the public.

Discussion Topics

1. Discuss the professional association's accountability to the profession and to society to set the standards for the profession.

2. Discuss the difference between this accountability by the professional association and the authority that the state nursing practice act has for determining practice.

3. Do you have access to the ANA Standards of Professional Nursing Practice in your organization? Where are they kept, is this convenient for the staff to access, and how could they be made more visible for the staff to use?

4. Choose specific Standards of Practice and Standards of Professional Performance, and compare the competencies for each with your evaluation tools.

5. *Reflection*—How can I increase my personal use of both the Standards of Practice and the Standards of Professional Performance? How could I encourage or model use of the standards to increase my colleagues' use of the standards?

References and Other Sources

American Nurses Association (ANA). (2001). *Code of Ethics for Nurses with interpretive statements*. Silver Spring, MD: Nursesbooks.org.

American Nurses Association (ANA). (2008). *Professional role competence.* Silver Spring, MD: Author. Retrieved from http://www.nursingworld.org/ MainMenuCategories/Policy-Advocacy/Positions-and-Resolutions/ ANAPositionStatements/Position-Statements-Alphabetically/ Professional-Role-Competence.html

American Nurses Association (ANA). (2009). *Nursing administration: Scope and standards of practice* (3rd ed.). Silver Spring, MD: Nursesbooks.org.

American Nurses Association (ANA). (2010a). *Nursing's social policy statement: The essence of the profession.* Silver Spring, MD: Nursesbooks.org.

American Nurses Association (ANA). (2010b). *Nursing: Scope and standards of practice* (2nd ed.). Silver Spring, MD: Nursesbooks.org.

American Nurses Association (ANA). (2010c). *Recognition of a nursing specialty, approval of a specialty nursing scope of practice statement, and acknowledgment of specialty nursing standards of practice.* Silver Spring, MD: Author.

American Nurses Credentialing Center (ANCC). (2012). Magnet Recognition Program®: Program overview. Retrieved from http://www.nursecredentialing .org/Magnet/ProgramOverview.aspx

Drenkard, K., Wolf, G., & Morgan, S. (2011). *Magnet®: The next generation— Nurses making the difference.* Silver Spring, MD: American Nurses Credentialing Center, Magnet Recognition Program®.

Hall, R. (1968). Professionalization and bureaucratization. *American Sociological Review, 33*(1), 92–104.

Houle, C. (1980). *Continuing learning in the professions.* San Francisco: Jossey-Bass.

Merton, R. (1958). The functions of the professional association. *The American Journal of Nursing, 58*(1), 50–54.

CHAPTER 4
Standard 1. Assessment

Sharon J. Olsen, PhD, RN, AOCN

***Standard 1. Assessment.* The registered nurse collects comprehensive data pertinent to the healthcare consumer's health and/or the situation.**

Definition and Explanation of the Standard

Assessment is the foundation on which all health promotion, risk reduction for disease, prevention of illness and injury, care management, and organizational decision-making is built. Systematic and continuous data collection establishes a basis for the clinical reasoning necessary to respond to changes in an effective and timely manner. The use of valid and reliable assessment tools for documentation promotes the collection of a standardized set of information. Further, such tools support a shared understanding of information across disciplines, promote the comparison of data, and enhance data dissemination via electronic pathways within and across organizations. Because nurses are continuously at the bedside or may be the first and often only health professional to see an individual in the community, assessment skills must be practiced and refined to a high level.

Data Collection

Assessment, a requisite skill of nurses at all levels of academic preparation, is the collection of "comprehensive data pertinent to the healthcare consumer's health and/or the situation" (ANA, 2010, p. 9). Typical data include but are not limited to the following domains: age, cognitive, cultural, economic, emotional, environmental, functional, organizational, physical, psychosocial, sexual, spiritual, and transpersonal.

Assessment is contextual. The type and amount of emergent data collected on a patient with a life-threatening gunshot wound in a fast-paced Level 1 trauma center will differ from that collected from an elderly patient who underwent a hip replacement and is being considered for discharge to home or a long-term care facility. The latter will additionally necessitate assessment of financial, family, and community resources, as well as the need for environmental accommodations in the home.

The relevance of context extends to role. For example, following transition from one shift to the next, an oncoming staff nurse will typically make patient rounds to conduct a brief assessment of patient status and to update the plan of care. This type of repetitive physical assessment provides the opportunity to anticipate or identify evolving changes in status. For the nurse manager, recurring errors drive the need to analyze outcome data for contributing factors and to review the literature for relevant interventions to change practice and improve quality of care. Nurse educators must assess not only *how* but also *what* staff nurses teach. Relevant data include the following:

- Existing clinical knowledge (assessed via survey, observed performance, or outcome data).

- Information on literacy (standardized tools are available that not only assess human literacy but also assess the literacy level of written materials).

- Age, gender, developmental, and ethnic differences in learning styles and values.

- Availability of materials in diverse languages.

Assessment is a continuous and iterative process driven by responses. The types and frequency of data collected from a patient with second-degree burns over 25% of his or her body changes over time and are analyzed differently. For example, an immediate goal may be pain relief requiring frequent assessments for adequate and sustained pain management. Over time, concerns about body image, physical function, and discharge to home will take on new urgency and will require the collection of broader types of information to secure appropriate interventions for those evolving issues.

Assessment varies according to the education and expertise of each nurse. Whereas new nurse graduates tend to think more linearly and to conduct assessments that are driven by tools with standardized parameters (e.g., instruments that measure fatigue, cognitive status, performance status, etc.), the graduate-level prepared specialty nurse and advanced practice registered nurse (APRN) are expected to critique the reliability and validity of assessment tools and to recognize gaps necessitating the addition, adaptation, or development of more contextually relevant tools that may be better suited to existing patient conditions, co-morbidities, or culture, as well as the changing demands of an organization for more technologically relevant assessment options.

Finally, assessment knowledge and skill requirements will change in relation to the demands of society, the need to translate new research into practice, and the changes in the dynamics of the healthcare system. One example concerns the rapid growth in society's understanding the relevance of cancer genetics and genomics for individualized risk assessment and the use of this information to guide decision-making around genetic testing and the use of targeted biologic treatments. In this instance, the cutting-edge nurse of today is expected to collect sufficient data to elicit a three-generation family health history and to construct a pedigree from this information using standardized symbols. The information can then be used to identify individuals at increased risk for disease and possible candidates for referral for genetic counseling. The graduate-level prepared specialty nurse and APRN would be expected to collaborate with genetic counselors and other specialists to develop and implement a plan of care that incorporates the genetic and genomic assessment information (Consensus Panel on Genetic/Genomic Nursing Competencies, 2009, p. 12).

A second example concerns the more contemporary focus on patient- and family-centered care. Whereas all nurses must ensure that patient and family values, preferences, expressed needs, and knowledge of the healthcare situation are considered in treatment planning, the graduate-level prepared specialty nurse and APRN may additionally examine the appropriateness of existing models of patient-centered care for selective use in particular units, departments, or organizations.

Synthesis

In the nursing process, assessment includes not only data collection but also synthesis of that data. Synthesis combines data elements to construct a coherent whole. All nurses are expected to synthesize complex information and to identify and prioritize problems and trends. Then nurses are expected to use the information to plan, provide, and direct care that maximizes health outcomes for patients and families; to improve knowledge and skills among staff members; and to enhance organizational capacity to provide safe, high-quality, and cost-effective care. At the heart of synthesis is a foundation of formal theoretical and scientific knowledge that is informed by experiential knowledge garnered from exposure to many particular clinical situations (Benner, Sutphen, Leonard, & Day, 2009). One's background frames what is attended to and how data are prioritized. Hence, nurses with greater experience and advanced education are expected to be able to recognize and efficiently correct gaps in information, to recognize salient data and trends, and to apply theoretical models in ways that enhance their ability to enable rapid and highly targeted responses to patient, practice, and organizational problems.

Application of the Standard in Practice

Education

Nursing students should receive structured and systematic teaching and evaluation of clinical assessment skills. Current nursing education programs facilitate this process in both academic and clinical environments. The use of laboratory options for student-to-student interviewing and physical assessment, the use of simulation technology, and the use of volunteer patients or "standardized patients" (often for intimate physical examinations) allow learners to practice, make mistakes, and learn from their mistakes without patients suffering adverse clinical consequences. The use of laboratory options, simulation technology, and volunteer patients also offers more control over the learning experience. However, transferring this learning to real patients requires that educators attend to such factors as similarity of physical characteristics between the learning and the practice settings, approximation of sensory stimuli, and ability to maximize students' perception that the simulation is a surrogate for the real experience (Teteris, Fraser, Wright, & McLaughlin, 2011). The use of standardized patients, though expensive, can smooth the bridge between simulation and clinical practice settings, as well as offer invaluable real-time guidance and feedback on student skills (Jha, Setna, Al-Hity, Quinton, & Roberts, 2010).

Educators typically provide standardized formats for the systematic collection of patient data, but students need guidance in selecting and prioritizing relevant data. Nursing students need to learn to draw valid conclusions from a set of data. Educators teach critical thinking skills as the means to assess and prioritize information before acting, and they give novice nursing students clear-cut rules to guide the analysis of the data. As nurses garner experience, they come to use intuition (the immediate recognition of patterns) to assist them in prioritizing and collecting data. Some graduate-level prepared specialty nurses and APRNs need to know how to initiate and interpret tests and procedures as part of the assessment process to prioritize medical diagnoses and justify medical and nursing plans of care.

Administration

Whereas a significant component of nursing assessment is patient- and family-focused, professional nurses who function as nurse administrators use the nursing process to shape policy; to develop strategic plans for nursing practice and care; to guide organizational, departmental, and unit-based initiatives; and to advocate for nursing systems that improve quality and provide excellence in care (ANA, 2009). Each of these actions must begin with an in-depth assessment and identification of the factors contributing to the potential or specific problem.

As with most nurses, nurse administrators make decisions based on evidence and data. Because relevant data in this case must often be drawn from many sources, clinicians as well as other stakeholders need to collect the data. Typically, nurse administrators synthesize clinical, human resource, risk-benefit, financial, quality, and regulatory data to identify patterns and variances. Sources of such data are generally standardized to allow benchmarking of outcomes across similar types and sizes of organizations (e.g., databases such as the National Database of Nursing Quality Indicators® [NDNQI®], the Healthcare Cost and Utilization Project databases, the Hospital Consumer Assessment of Healthcare Providers and Systems [HCAPS] data, and patient satisfaction surveys [Gallup, Press Ganey]).

Performance and Quality Improvement

Quality assurance programs are designed to analyze healthcare requirements and to determine ways of ensuring that protocols and standards are followed. The programs include a system to audit requisite standards for compliance through the assessment of physiologic, psychosocial, functional, and operational outcomes data and the ability to institute performance improvement plans when standards are not met. Nurses are critical stakeholders in these programs. And nurses at all levels are professionally accountable for ensuring that the care they provide improves patient outcomes. Standards of practice, protocols, and practice guidelines promote evidence-driven care. The continuous and prospective analysis of patient outcomes that correlate with nursing behaviors can be gathered and generated to determine areas of progress and deficiency using data systematically recorded in the NDNQI database. Graduate-level prepared specialty nurses and APRNs are expected to regularly assess the practice environment for potential risks to patient safety, autonomy, and quality of care (National CNS Competency Task Force, 2010). These data can identify the need for new and revised programs or the development of new healthcare standards that will be based on evidence.

Research

Nurses are expected to provide care that is driven by evidence (Evidence-Based Practice [EBP]) to ensure optimal clinical outcomes and quality of life. In the face of new or recurring clinical problems, the first step in EBP is assessment and should include a critical appraisal of the factors associated with the problem, a survey of the patient's knowledge and values associated with the problem, and a rigorous analysis of the published literature.

Assessment can take on other aspects in research. For example, one might assess the research competencies of nurses, assess *health status* as part of a research hypothesis, or use an assessment tool to garner data to answer research questions. A couple of examples follow.

According to Galassi et al. (in progress), "nursing practice is informed by evidence, evidence comes from research, research leads to improved health outcomes, and research findings should guide nursing practice." In their assessment of the research competencies of nurses who have earned a bachelor of science in nursing, the study discovered that nurses were poorly prepared to lead clinical research or clinical trials and, consequently, poorly qualified to educate patients about these tasks. Drawing on this assessment, the authors provided recommendations for academic coursework in clinical research and clinical trials and went on to publish professional competencies that set the expectation that clinical research is a professional responsibility of master's prepared nurses.

In another example, Thomas Ahrens, a critical care nurse and physiologist, noted the "availability of new and more accurate assessment techniques has been slow to be adopted by clinicians," thus citing the fact that "current vital signs are more than 100 years old, and they are misleading and often inaccurate" as an example of the need to improve the "practice of bedside monitoring" and the need to ground assessment in scientific evidence and move it beyond dogma (in Benner, Hooper-Kyriakidis, & Stannard 2011).

The work of O'Conaire, Rushton, and Wright (2011) is instructive in this area. The aim of their study was to assess the inter-rater reliability and precision of a novel device to improve use of a tuning fork and to evaluate its concurrent validity with a Vibrameter®. Those tools are used to assess vibration sense during a musculoskeletal exam. The researchers concluded that the tuning fork and novel device demonstrated a strong correlation with the Vibrameter. There was good concurrent validity and moderate inter-rater reliability among healthy subjects, but the authors recommended further study with affected subjects.

Using valid and reliable assessment tools for documentation promotes the collection of a standardized set of information. Nurses must ensure that evidence-based assessment techniques are used in the clinical environment. Whereas all nurses can be involved in data collection for clinical research, graduate-level prepared specialty nurses and APRNs can be expected to design and implement similar assessment studies and to educate staff nurses in deficiency areas that are necessary to participate more broadly in research studies.

Conclusion

Standard 1 Assessment describes the expectation that the registered nurse collects comprehensive data pertinent to the health and environment of healthcare consumers. This essential and foundational first step in the nursing process demands competency in the collection, synthesis, and critical appraisal of available clinical and published data about the healthcare consumer as well as the family, family dynamics, and context of care. Evidence-based assessment incorporates recognition of the values, preferences, and expressed needs of healthcare consumers, who are the ultimate authorities on their own health.

Case Study and Discussion Topics

The following case provides examples of how assessment might change over time and how it might vary by professional role.

Case Study

Ms. Alexander is a 51-year-old married woman who has mild hypertension and obesity and who was recently diagnosed with Stage II breast cancer. She has a paternal history of breast and ovarian cancer.

ASSESSMENT

All RNs should be able to do the following:

- Identify the types of information and standard assessment tool(s) you might use to determine eligibility for referral to a genetic counselor.

- Discuss any ethical, legal, or privacy implications of accessing genetic information.

- Identify the types of information necessary to garner an accurate assessment of the psychological and social resources your patient needs to cope with this diagnosis.

Nurses prepared for advanced clinical and managerial roles should be able to do the following:

- Identify contextual and etiologic assessment data (including both non-disease-related and disease-related factors) necessary to formulate differential diagnoses.

- Critically assess the relevance of national standards for recommending a plan of care.

- Suggest data that should be recorded and tracked to assess patient responses to treatment.

Case continued . . . Ms. Alexander underwent a mastectomy with four axillary nodes resected. Radiation therapy consisting of postoperative external-beam radiation therapy to the entire breast was completed over five weeks. She subsequently received chemotherapy with doxorubicin and cyclophosphamide and will continue on tamoxifen for five years. Possible late toxic effects of radiation therapy, though uncommon, can include radiation pneumonitis, cardiac events, lymphedema, brachial plexopathy, and the risk of second malignancies. Side effects associated with tamoxifen include endometrial cancer, DVT (deep vein thrombosis), and PE (pulmonary embolism).

ASSESSMENT
All RNs should be able to do the following:

- Identify data that can be used to assess the patient's knowledge and perceptions of her treatment and her ability to identify salient effects of therapy that should be reported to the medical oncologist, radiation oncologist, and primary care provider.

Nurses prepared for advanced clinical and managerial roles should be able to do the following:

- Identify the sources and types of information you would need to develop an evidence-based lymphedema prevention program. You **should** do this **as an interprofessional team effort** in your practice knowing that there is no agreed-upon standard for guiding women who undergo breast cancer treatment about how to prevent lymphedema.

Case continued . . . Ms. Alexander is now three years post-treatment. As Ms. Alexander's primary care provider, you, the nurse practitioner, recognize that cancer survivors have needs that are often better addressed by non-oncology practitioners, but this coordination requires that all stakeholders (oncologists, primary care providers, and patients) acknowledge, accept, and coordinate the efforts. National data on patterns of preventive care among breast cancer survivors have shown that breast cancer survivors are less likely to receive preventive care services, such as flu shots, cholesterol screening, and colorectal cancer screening, compared with non-cancer controls. However, survivors managed by both a primary care provider and an oncology specialist were more likely to receive appropriate care. You are also aware that recent studies of postmenopausal breast cancer survivors show higher risks of death from cardiovascular disease than from breast cancer.

ASSESSMENT

All RNs should be able to do the following:

- Specify the physical and lifestyle data you would need to gather to determine needs for patient education about disease prevention and screening on the basis of national guidelines for disease prevention and screening for a 54-year-old woman.

Nurses prepared for advanced clinical and managerial roles should be able to do the following:

- Prioritize health history and physical exam findings to develop individualized, age-appropriate disease prevention and screening follow-up care plans.

- Recognize that there is a lack of data about the long-term effects of treatment on breast cancer survivors. Discuss the need to implement changes in systems that promote the assessment and tracking of outcome indicators of breast cancer survivor status.

References and Other Sources

American Nurses Association (ANA). (2009). *Nursing administration: Scope and standards of practice.* Silver Spring, MD: Nursesbooks.org.

American Nurses Association (ANA). (2010). *Nursing: Scope and standards of practice* (2nd ed.). Silver Spring, MD: Nursesbooks.org.

Benner, P., Hooper-Kyriakidis, P., & Stannard, D. (2011) *Clinical wisdom and interventions in acute and critical care: A thinking-in-action approach* (2nd ed.). New York: Springer Publishing Co.

Benner, P., Sutphen, M., Leonard, V., & Day, L. (2009). *Educating nurses: A call for radical transformation.* San Francisco: Jossey Bass.

Consensus Panel on Genetic/Genomic Nursing Competencies. (2009). *Essentials of genetic and genomic nursing: Competencies, curricula guidelines, and outcome indicators* (2nd ed.). Silver Spring, MD: American Nurses Association.

Galassi, A., Grady, M., Parreco, L., Ness, E., O'Mara, A., Hastings, C., Browning, S., & Belcher, A. (2011). *Changing the culture: Clinical research, clinical trials (CR/CT), and baccalaureate nursing education.* Bethesda, MD: National Institutes of Health, National Cancer Institute. Retrieved from https://ccrod.cancer.gov/confluence/download/attachments/78384884/Grand_Rounds_09_28_11.pdf?version=1&modificationDate=1331323356683

Jha, V., Setna, Z., Al-Hity, A., Quinton, N. D., & Roberts, T. E. (2010). Patient involvement in teaching and assessing intimate examination skills: A systematic review. *Medical Education, 44,* 347–357.

National CNS Competency Task Force. (2010). *Clinical nurse specialist core competencies: Executive summary 2006–2008.* Philadelphia: National Association of Clinical Nurse Specialists.

O'Conaire, E., Rushton, A., & Wright, C. (2011). The assessment of vibration sense in the musculoskeletal examination: Moving towards a valid and reliable quantitative approach to vibration testing in clinical practice. *Manual Therapy, 16*(3), 296–300.

Teteris, E., Fraser, K., Wright, B., & McLaughlin, K. (June 2011). Does training learners on simulators benefit real patients? *Advances in Health Science Education.* doi:10.1007/s10459-011-9304-5.

U.S. Department of Health and Human Services. (2002). *Nurse practitioner primary care competencies in specialty areas: Adult, family, gerontological, pediatric, and women's health.* Rockville, MD: Health Resources and Services Administration, Bureau of Health Professions, Division of Nursing.

CHAPTER 5

Standard 2. Diagnosis

Julie Stanik-Hutt, PhD, ACNP-BC, CCNS, FAAN

Standard 2. Diagnosis. **The registered nurse analyzes the assessment data to determine the diagnosis or the issues.**

Definition and Explanation of the Standard

Diagnosis refers to the process of critically evaluating an issue or situation to identify and apply a name to the cause of the problem (Merriam-Webster Online Dictionary, 2011). Diagnostic processes are used by individuals in many occupations and professions. In addition to healthcare professionals, many others, including engineers, teachers, managers, automobile mechanics, and plumbers, diagnose problems within their areas of expertise. Healthcare professionals use the diagnostic process to identify and name the most likely cause of a patient's signs and symptoms (Rakel, 2011). To make a diagnosis, the healthcare provider uses clinical judgment to draw conclusions regarding the nature or cause of the health problem on the basis of the available data. These problems, labeled as diagnoses, become the focus for planning care. In clinical practice, nurses use diagnosis to determine and name individual patient's health problems. Nurses also use diagnosis to identify and name healthcare systems problems that interfere with effective delivery of high-quality healthcare services. In either case, the nurse recognizes a deviation from the expected, collects information about the deviation, interprets and analyses the assessment data, draws a conclusion, and labels the problem. Diagnosis is the second step of the nursing process.

Diagnoses serve several purposes. In clinical practice, diagnoses are used to identify a patient's problems, which are the focus of attention by the health-care provider. On the basis of that diagnosis, the provider develops a plan of care with established goals and selected effective therapeutic interventions. Diagnoses also facilitate communication among healthcare providers. By using standard diagnostic terms, multiple healthcare providers can understand the patient's problems, can anticipate interventions that will be used to manage the problem, and can expect that certain data will be collected to reassess the patient's condition and responses to care (Muller-Staub, Lavin, Needham, & van Achterberg, 2006). Diagnostic language can also be used as a system to organize research and practice evaluation processes, and it can be used to create a system of nomenclature for reimbursement for healthcare services (Rutherford, 2008).

Types of Diagnoses Used in Nursing

The type of diagnostic language used by nurses differentiates the practice focus of nursing and their professional role from those of other healthcare providers. Registered nurses (RNs) use nursing diagnoses to characterize and organize their professional work. In contrast, medical diagnoses label genetic and pathological conditions, illnesses, and syndromes. Medical diagnoses are used by APRNs nurse practitioners (NPs), nurse anesthetists (CRNAs), clinical nurse specialists (CNSs), physicians, nurse midwives (CNMs), and some other healthcare providers. Nurses in leadership and executive positions (clinical nurse specialists, nurse managers, nurse executives, nurse educators) also use critical thinking and problem-solving processes to identify and label (diagnose) problems that they encounter in their work. Although they may not always use a set of standardized diagnostic terms or labels, they are using similar processes to move from assessment of a situation to identification of a cause(s) before developing a plan of action to resolve or correct the problem.

A nursing diagnosis is defined as an actual or potential response to a health problem experienced by a patient, family, or community, including health promotion needs and risks for health problems and syndromes. The North American Nursing Diagnosis Association International (NANDA-I) is one orga-nization that has developed a diagnostic language commonly used in nursing. NANDA-I diagnoses are commonly used with two associated compendia, the Nursing Interventions Classifications (NIC) (Bulechek, Butcher, & Dochterman, 2008) and the Nursing Outcomes Classifications (NOC) (Moorhead, Johnson, Maas, & Swanson, 2007). The International Classification of Nursing Practice

(ICNP) and Perioperative Nursing Data Set (PNDS) are two other systems used to label patient healthcare problems addressed through nursing (ICN, 2009; Peterson, 2011). All three of these systems (NANDA-I with NIC and NOC, ICNP, and PNDS) integrate diagnostic terminology with nursing interventions and expected outcomes.

Within the NANDA-I system, each diagnostic term includes a definition statement (diagnostic criteria), related factors (etiology of the problem, contributing or associated factors), and defining characteristics (symptoms) (Ackley & Ladwig, 2011). Consequently, a NANDA-I nursing diagnosis includes three parts: the problem, the etiology of the problem, and the symptoms. For example, a patient who has coronary artery disease and who grimaces and complains of 7/10 burning pain while pointing to the middle of his or her chest might have the nursing diagnosis of acute pain related to myocardial ischemia as evidenced by patient's grimace and complaint of 7/10 burning pain. The information provided in the NANDA-I fully describes the diagnosis of interest. Categories included in the NANDA-I system include physical, psychological, sociocultural, and spiritual responses to health problems. The Omaha System and the Clinical Care Classification System also identify health problems and interventions used by nurses (Martin, 2005; Saba, 2006). The Omaha System includes categories for several domains: environmental, psychological, physiological, and health behaviors. It is commonly used by nurses in home health and public health settings. The Clinical Care Classification System includes diagnoses and interventions originally designed for nurses to use to describe and document home health care.

A medical diagnosis is used to label genetic or pathological conditions, illnesses, and syndromes. Advanced practice registered nurses (APRNs) are legally authorized to make medical diagnoses. Diagnostic criteria used to make medical diagnoses consist of the patient symptoms, physical and psychological examination findings, and results on selected diagnostic tests. Diagnostic labels used are found in the *International Classification of Diseases* (ICD) and the *Diagnostic and Statistical Manual of Mental Disorders* (DSM) (WHO, 2007; American Psychiatric Association, 2000). The ICD is a taxonomy of diagnostic language used in medical diagnosis. It includes an exhaustive list of diagnoses and patient symptoms, signs, and injuries. The DSM is another system of diagnostic language used in medicine. It includes diagnostic criteria for and the standard diagnostic terminology used by all providers (NPs, psychiatric clinical nurse specialists [CNSs], MDs, psychologists, etc.) to identify psychiatric and mental health problems.

Two other systems, the International Classification of Functioning, Disability, and Health (ICF) and the Systematized Nomenclature of Medicine—Clinical Terms (SNOMED CT) are used with diagnostic languages, primarily to organize research and practice evaluation processes (WHO, 2011; Ruch, Gobeill, Lovis, & Geissbühler, 2008). The ICF system classifies "health and disability at both individual and population levels" (WHO, 2011). It is used alongside medical diagnostic language to describe an individual's functional capacities, including performance of activities of daily living as well as one's ability to interact with others. The ICF is not used in clinical practice in the United States, although it is used in Australia and Italy "to document functional status assessment, goal setting, and treatment planning and monitoring, as well as outcome measurement" (WHO, 2011). The ICF has been used more widely to describe the health status of a country's population.

SNOMED CT is an exhaustive system of highly refined and technically specific clinical language used in clinical information systems to code, retrieve, and analyze information related to healthcare encounters. The system is integrated in such a way that varying labels for the same problem are linked. In this way, searches will retrieve all relevant cases so that care processes and outcomes can be examined. Although SNOMED CT includes diagnostic labels, it also includes much more specific technical terminology that is not generally used in practice to make nursing or medical diagnoses.

The Diagnostic Process

PATIENT-FOCUSED CARE

Assessment data (symptoms and physical exam findings) are the defining characteristics (diagnostic criteria) used to narrow the broad list of potential diagnoses to the one that is or ones that are the best match to the patient's situation. More than one diagnosis may match the patient's symptoms. After collecting assessment data, the nurse analyzes the patient's historical data, symptoms, and physical examination findings are and organizes them into related groups or categories. A patient's symptoms and signs can be grouped to create a cohesive picture of all associated data. For example, during the assessment process, a patient who complains of difficulty breathing would be asked questions that would further describe the symptom (e.g., onset, duration, and aggravating factors), and he or she would be examined for physical evidence related to breathing difficulty (e.g., respiratory rate and pattern, oximetry readings, breath sounds, color, and diaphoresis). All those data are analyzed together to identify the diagnoses related to the patient's complaint of difficulty breathing. Whenever possible, diagnoses are validated with the patient, family, or community (American Nurses Association, 2010; pg. 34).

POPULATION-FOCUSED CARE

When an individual patient and his or her family are the focus in community-based care, nursing assessment and diagnoses are used as they are with any other individual or family (Rivera & Parris, 2002). When working with a community, a diagnosis is based on data from a focused or comprehensive community health assessment while using population-based health data, socio-economic and crime statistics, data about family makeup and cultural groups, and the physical characteristics as well as the safety of the environment. The "10 Essential Public Health Services" might also be used to inform collection and analysis of assessment data (Public Health Functions Steering Committee, 1994; Smith & Bazini-Barakat, 2003; Satterfield, et al., 2004). Data from all these diverse sources are organized and analyzed to identify population-based health problems. Relevant diagnoses might include items such as ineffective community coping and health maintenance; risk prone behavior for injury and trauma, for poisoning, for impaired parenting, and similar items; deficient knowledge related to readiness for enhanced self-health management; social isolation; and so forth.

SYSTEMS OF CARE

Nurse executives, CNSs, and clinical educators engage in identifying and labeling other problems within healthcare organizations and systems. Although the problems might not be called diagnoses, their identification is preceded by the same process and is followed by the same steps of planning, implementation, and evaluation. Areas that might be assessed include care systems, quality and safety, finance, communications, patient satisfaction, regulatory issues, personnel, organizational culture and space, and equipment and supply resources. Assessment data would come from a variety of sources, such as unit, departmental, and system-wide staffing patterns; staff knowledge and skill levels; patient satisfaction surveys; unit performance on safety or quality indicators; and human resource data, such as data on retention and work-related injuries.

Diagnoses might include the use of some nursing diagnostic language, as well as other types of language, to identify problems. For example, the following three nursing diagnoses might apply: (1) deficient knowledge related to new medical diagnosis and new medication regimen_____, (2) readiness to learn, parenting skills, related to birth of first baby_____, or (3) risk for injury; hematoma: risk factor related to invasive procedure. Other diagnostic terms might refer to the need to improve interprofessional or inter-unit communications, the need to improve patient satisfaction related to timeliness of staff responses to a request for assistance (call bell time), and the need to decrease medication error rates in general or related to late administration.

LAW AND REGULATION

Scope of practice, practice authority, and legal boundaries for NPs, CRNAs, and CNMs differ from those of RNs. All RNs are legally authorized to make nursing diagnoses. In addition, NPs, CRNAs, and CNMs use differential diagnostic processes to independently make medical diagnoses (National Organization of Nurse Practitioner Faculties, 2006; AANA, 2010; American College of Nurse Midwives, 2009). Graduate prepared specialty nurses and APRNs are authorized to diagnose and manage medical problems, to prescribe medications and therapies, to order and interpret diagnostic tests, and to receive direct reimbursement for "physician" services that they provide. In contrast, the scope of practice, practice authority, and legal boundaries of CNSs, APHNs, and NEs in general do not differ from those of RNs.

The act of making a medical diagnosis carries legal implications beyond those associated with the use of a nursing diagnosis. A medical diagnosis defines the pathological or genetic cause of a health problem. Once that label is applied, it can subsequently be used by insurance actuaries to estimate life expectancy and risk for future healthcare problems. Missed medical diagnoses can result in treatment delays or omissions, which can result in permanent disability and even death. Consequently, use of an incorrect medical diagnosis can lead to legal action if a patient is harmed or if the diagnostician is not legally authorized. As such, medical diagnoses should be used only by legally authorized individuals when diagnostic criteria have been met.

ADVANCED PRACTICE REGISTERED NURSING

Several methods are used to reach a final medical diagnosis. The first approach for commonly encountered diagnoses is the *pattern matching* approach. It involves the recognition of a set of signs and symptoms to represent a pattern associated with a specific diagnosis. This method relies on the provider's experience, a consistent set of presentation patterns for the disease, and the provider's recognition of the pattern. An example of the use of pattern matching would be immediate recognition of serous otitis media in a 12-year-old patient who presents complaining of mild ear pain without fever and who has a history of a recent upper respiratory infection. Because patients do not present with consistent clinical findings for most diagnoses, pattern recognition does not provide consistently accurate results.

In the second method, which is used in most situations, providers approach the diagnostic process systematically. They develop a list of potential (differential) diagnoses while being sure to avoid omitting any potential pathological causes that might be causing a patient's signs and symptoms. Then providers use the *hypothesis testing* method (a deductive reasoning approach) to work through the list of possible diagnoses—systematically eliminating those that do not match assessment data—until a final diagnostic conclusion is reached. The providers use clinical judgment and a systematic process while "comparing and contrasting the clinical findings, to determine which of the potential diagnoses is the one from which the patient is suffering" (*Stedman's Medical Dictionary*, 2006, p. 492). For example, angina (cardiac ischemia) is a diagnosis immediately suspected when a middle-aged patient presents with the symptom of chest pain, especially if it is associated with shortness of breath, lightheadedness, nausea, and diaphoresis. However, the provider would consider other potential diagnoses related to structures in the chest and systems that could produce chest pain, including cardiovascular, pulmonary, gastrointestinal, and musculoskeletal. This approach would produce a list of suspected diagnoses, including pericarditis, aortic dissection, pulmonary embolism, tension pneumothorax, pneumonia, esophageal rupture, gastroesophageal reflux disease, and costochondritis. Although angina might be the working decision, the provider would collect and analyze more data to eliminate other diagnoses on the differential list and to confirm that the working diagnosis is the true diagnosis.

The third approach to medical diagnosis includes using decision trees or algorithms to work through the potential causes of a sign or symptom. Algorithms allow the provider to systematically proceed through a series of decision points to reach a final diagnosis. At each step in the algorithm, the provider answers a yes or no question about the patient's assessment data. Each item of relevant assessment data is considered as the algorithm is used, and diagnoses that do not match the data are eliminated. When using the *differential diagnosis* or *algorithmic* approach, the provider usually identifies an initial working diagnosis early. A working diagnosis is a provisional diagnosis that is most likely believed to be the true diagnosis. Use of a working diagnosis allows the provider to initiate a therapeutic plan while further diagnostic work proceeds. The plan is often revised when additional diagnostic information becomes available. The final diagnosis will not be made until all other potential diagnoses have been excluded (ruled out) and the true diagnosis has been confirmed (ruled in).

Application of the Standard in Practice

Education

Professional nurses are educated to design and deliver nursing care to individuals, families, and communities (AACN, 2008). To do so, nursing students are taught the nursing process and provided opportunities to apply each of the steps of the nursing process (assessment, diagnosis, planning, implementation, and evaluation) during clinical experiences. Nursing diagnosis is emphasized in basic nursing education. Students are taught about NANDA-I, the Omaha System, and other diagnostic and care planning systems (for example, NIC and NOC). Students learn to use nursing diagnosis to direct patient care and to evaluate the outcomes of that care. Through nursing diagnosis, students learn to understand the discipline of nursing, nursing's unique role in health care, and the scope of professional nursing practice. Problem-focused learning and problem-based teaching foster the development of students' skills in critical thinking. CNSs, with their dual preparation as experts in nursing and as nurse educators, are ideally suited to assist nursing students acquire diagnostic skills and apply those skills to complex cases.

Nurses pursuing graduate education in advanced nursing complete didactic instruction and clinical learning experiences to master the competencies related to the specialty and the advanced nursing practice role to which they aspire. Diagnosis is a prominent feature of advanced nursing practice. Problem-based learning predominates in those programs, and students apply expanded skills, including new diagnostic skills, to real patient situations under the tutelage of APRNs and others (e.g., physicians, healthcare administrators, and public health practitioners) with relevant healthcare skills. NPs, CRNAs, CNMs, and APRNs learn to make medical diagnosis during their graduate education. They demonstrate competency in medical diagnosis during supervised clinical experiences and certification examinations. CNS students acquire additional skills in the diagnosis of systems problems that impede high-quality care. For example, CNSs diagnose knowledge deficits among nursing personnel and other healthcare providers. Advanced nurse executives, along with CNSs, diagnose a variety of unit- and systems-level problems (inadequate staffing or staff mix, communications, resource distribution, and other care process problems) that produce barriers to high-quality, safe patient care (NACNS, 2009; National CNS Competency Task Force, 2010; AONE, 2005). They also diagnose broader problems that impede effective operation of healthcare delivery systems (e.g., population variables, environmental and political issues, and regulatory and financial issues). Graduate-level public health nurses (also called advanced public health nurses, or APHNs) are expected to apply advanced knowledge of nursing and public health to diagnose population- and systems-related health problems (ACHNE, 2007).

Administration

The application of diagnosis in the design, organization, and implementation of direct patient care has already been described. Diagnosis also provides a basis for documentation of the type of problems and care required by individuals and groups of patients. Administrators find this documentation useful in making decisions about grouping patients, selecting care models, creating nursing personnel mix, acquiring needed ancillary resources, and using capital equipment and disposables. Using a standard language to document diagnoses helps nurse administrators evaluate care provided to groups of patients with the same diagnosis. It allows care quality for the group to be evaluated and to be compared to care at other institutions. Then, it allows quality improvement initiatives to be implemented. When administrators use standard diagnostic terms, they find those terms facilitate their use of information technologies to retrieve aggregated data by diagnosis for planning, analysis, and interpretation of healthcare data.

Performance and Quality Improvement

Many diagnoses and systems problems commonly encountered in nursing practice are targets for quality improvement. Higher priority attention is usually given to diagnoses or problems that are associated with increased risk, cost, or volume. For example, ineffective interprofessional communication of the patient's needs and of plans at patient transitions is commonly identified or diagnosed as a problem within a healthcare system and can benefit from quality improvement activities. Disruptive communications and behaviors is another priority factor that has been added to regulators' quality standards for systems (Joint Commission, 2008). Personnel knowledge deficits, risk of patient injury, ineffective decision-making, hospital-acquired infections, and other problems are also systems diagnoses that might be addressed through quality improvement. Many quality measures associated with specific patient diagnoses are used in practice improvement initiatives. Those measures include controlling high blood pressure in diabetes, using oral antiplatelet medications in coronary artery disease, discontinuing prophylactic antibiotics within 24 hours of surgery, screening women over 64 for osteoporosis, and many others (Centers for Medicare and Medicaid, 2011).

Research

Having nurses proficiently use standard diagnostic language is important for developing nursing's unique body of knowledge, as well as for assessing the effect of nursing on health care in general. When providers use standard diagnostic language, data from patients with the same diagnoses can be aggregated for analysis and interpretation. Standard language is also critical for developing information systems (e.g., SNOMED CT) and their capacity to provide an adequate legal record of care; for developing and applying relevant clinical decision support systems; for capturing nursing's financial contribution to health care; and for developing databases that can be used for clinical administrative, quality improvement, and research activities (Zielstorff, 1998; Westra, 2005). The use of a standard set of diagnoses, especially when linked to interventions and outcomes evaluation, is critical to generate and disseminate research and quality improvement data. Those data are important to policy decision-making not only within healthcare organizations and associated groups (e.g., insurance providers), but also within government agencies. Use of a standard diagnostic language is critical to nursing's research and policy agendas and to the translation of research into practice in order to enhance care and patient outcomes.

Conclusion

Standard 2 Diagnosis describes the expectation that the registered nurse obtains and analyzes assessment data to determine the diagnoses or the problem and uses appropriate terminology systems on the basis of level of education and legal authority. This second step in the nursing process requires the knowledge, skills, and ability to derive the diagnoses or problems from the available data and information, including the identification of actual or potential risks or barriers to health. Validation of the diagnoses or problems with the healthcare consumer, family, and other healthcare providers is an associated competency and helps prepare for the next step: identification of expected outcomes.

Case Studies and Discussion Topics

Case Study 1, Part 1

Mrs. Smith is a 75-year-old woman admitted after an abrupt syncopal episode on arising from the toilet after defecating. She awoke lying on the bathroom floor, got up, walked to a chair, and called 911. On her arrival at the Emergency Department, her Review of Systems was positive for (1) several days of shortness of breath over the past one to two weeks, (2) occasional palpitations, and (3) increased fatigue. Several months ago, she was admitted to the hospital with a non-ST-elevation myocardial infarction complicated by symptoms of heart failure. Her ejection fraction at that time was 26%, but over subsequent months of medical management it rose to 50%. Mrs. Smith lives with her 80-year-old husband, who is very concerned about his wife's condition and is repeatedly asking questions about her plan of care.

A CT scan of her head ruled out stroke, and a carotid ultrasound ruled out significant carotid stenosis. Electrocardiogram and cardiac enzymes ruled out myocardial infarction, and subsequent monitoring has revealed no dysrhythmias. Postural vital signs and physical exam ruled out hypovolemia. Laboratory results ruled out significant anemia. Today, she underwent a cardiac catheterization to evaluate her coronary perfusion and to obtain intracardiac pressure measurements. No significant stenoses were found to the coronaries, the left ventricular filling pressure was slightly elevated, and her ejection fraction was 42%. Mean pressure gradient across the aortic valve was 56 mm.

Mrs. Smith had no complaints at this time.

Her past medical history includes coronary artery disease, myocardial infarction, heart failure, hypertension, dyslipidemia, and chronic renal insufficiency (baseline creatinine 1.4).

Her physical examination revealed the following:

- Vital signs: Temperature = 37.4 °F, pulse = 71, blood pressure = 156/80, respiratory rate = 16.

- Transcutaneous oximetry = 96% on room air

- 24-hour intake/output = unknown/1,100, weight = 63.9 Kg

General: Frail appearing, pleasant, elderly female in no acute distress. Awake and oriented times 3 cooperative.

Head, Eyes, Ears, Nose, and Throat (HEENT)/Neck: Normocephalic, atraumatic. Symmetrical features. Pupils equally round and reactive to light and accommodation, external ocular movements intact. Tongue midline. Mucous membranes are pink. Sclera anicteric, Cranial Nerves II through XII grossly intact. Neck supple, thyroid smooth.

Respiratory: Unlabored respirations with bilateral equal expansion. Scattered fine crackles.

Cardiovascular: Regular rate and rhythm. Normal S2. S1 obliterated by grade III/VI systolic ejection murmur at 2nd intercostal space, right sternal border. S4 present. No rub. No jugular venous distention. 2+ bilateral radial and dorsalis pedis pulses.

Abdomen: Flat, normal, active bowel sounds, soft non-distended, non-tender. No organomegaly.

Extremities: Warm, no femoral bruits, no edema. Right femoral puncture site soft, non-tender, without drainage or ecchymosis. Moves all extremities with bilateral equal strength of 5+/5.

Analysis of the assessment data would start with differentiation of normal from abnormal findings.

A. *What are the pertinent assessment data, both historical and physical examination, that you would use to make a diagnosis?*

Pertinent historical and examination data include the following:

- Past medical history of coronary artery disease, myocardial infarction, heart failure, hypertension, dyslipidemia, and chronic renal insufficiency (baseline creatinine 1.4).

- Symptoms of abrupt syncopal episode, shortness of breath, palpitations, and increased fatigue.

- Pertinent positive physical findings of these: Blood pressure = 156/80, scattered fine crackles, presence of S4. S1 obliterated by grade III/VI systolic ejection murmur at 2nd intercostal space, right sternal border. Slightly elevated left ventricular filling pressure and ejection fraction of 42%.

Pertinent negative physical findings include these:

- Pulse = 71, respiratory rate = 16, transcutaneous oximetry = 96% on room air; awake and oriented times 3; unlabored respirations; regular rate and rhythm, no jugular venous distention, 2+ bilateral radial and dorsalis pedis pulses, warm extremities; no femoral bruits, no edema, and right femoral puncture site soft, non-tender without drainage or ecchymosis.

- No significant stenoses were found to the coronaries.

B. *What basic nursing diagnoses would you make?*

The data indicate that Mrs. Smith has several problems related to her cardio-vascular function, and the registered nurse caring for her makes the following nursing diagnoses on the basis of her current condition:

- Decreased cardiac output related to history of myocardial infarction, heart failure, and hypertension as evidenced by shortness of breath, a 10-pound weight gain, and increased fatigue, blood pressure = 156/80, scattered fine crackles, presence of S4.

- Risk for injury: hematoma: risk factor invasive procedure.

- Caregiver role strain related to anticipated care-giving activities.

- Risk for deficient knowledge related to new diagnosis of aortic stenosis, impending surgery, and new medications.

C. *If you are an advanced practice registered nurse, what medical diagno-ses would you make?*

The nurse practitioner who is managing Mrs. Smith makes the following medical diagnoses:

- Heart failure.

- Severe aortic stenosis.

- Stable coronary artery disease.

- Uncontrolled hypertension.

Cardiac surgical consult is obtained and plans are made for the woman to undergo aortic valve replacement in two weeks. She will be discharged home in the morning on two new antihypertensive medications, which have been started in the hospital.

The clinical nurse specialist—recognizing that Mrs. Smith and her husband are dealing with a new diagnosis and medications and that patients with heart failure are at high risk for readmission within 30 days of discharge from the hospital—makes the following diagnoses:

- Risk for ineffective interprofessional communication between inpatient and outpatient care providers related to the new diagnosis of aortic stenosis, plans for surgery, and new medication regimen.

Case Study, Part 2

- Using a population health perspective, what diagnoses might you consider to address needs of patients similar to Mrs. Smith in the community?

- What is the role of the CNS in this case, and what effect do you think the CNS's diagnosis could have on the patient's outcome?

- Explain why the diagnoses made by the RN and NP differ even though they are based on the same patient history and examination data.

- What diagnostic taxonomies could be used to identify patient problems and to develop plans of care for Mrs. Smith after she is discharged home?

References and Other Sources

Ackley, B., & Ladwig, G. (2011). *Nursing diagnosis handbook* (9th ed.). St. Louis, MO: Mosby Elsevier.

American Association of Colleges of Nursing (AACN). (2008). *The essentials of baccalaureate education for professional nursing practice.* Washington, DC: Author.

American Association of Nurse Anesthetists (AANA). (2010). *Scope and standards for nurse anesthesia practice.* Park Ridge, IL: Author. Retrieved from http://www.aana.com/resources2/professionalpractice/Documents/PPM%20Scope%20and%20Standards.pdf

American College of Nurse Midwives. (2009). *Standards for the practice of midwifery.* Silver Spring, MD: Author. Retrieved from http://www.midwife.org/ACNM/files/ccLibraryFiles/Filename/000000000270/Standards_for_Practice_of_Midwifery_12_09_001.pdf

American Nurses Association (ANA). (2010). *Nursing: Scope and standards of practice* (2nd ed.). Silver Spring, MD: Nursesbooks.org.

American Organization of Nurse Executives (AONE). (2005). *AONE nurse executive competencies.* Retrieved from http://www.aone.org/resources/leadership%20tools/nursecomp.shtml

American Psychiatric Association. (2000). *Diagnostic and statistical manual of mental disorders* (4th ed., text rev.). Washington, DC: American Psychiatric Association.

Association of Community Health Nursing Educators (ACHNE). (2007). *Graduate education for advanced practice public health nursing: At the crossroads.* Wheat Ridge, CO: Author. Retrieved from http://www.achne .org/files/public/GraduateEducationDocument.pdf

Bulechek, G., Butcher, H., & Dochterman, J. (2008). *Nursing interventions classification (NIC).* St. Louis, MO: Mosby Elsevier.

Centers for Medicare and Medicaid. (2011). 2011 Physician quality reporting system (physician quality reporting) measures list. Retrieved from https://www.cms.gov/PQRS/Downloads/2011_PhysQualRptg_ MeasuresList_033111.pdf

How to write a nursing diagnosis: http://www.youtube.com/ watch?v=JyAaQ5hILSs6

International Council of Nurses (ICN). (2009). *The international classification for nursing practice.* Geneva, Switzerland: ICN.

The Joint Commission. (2008). Behaviors that undermine a culture of safety. Sentinel event alert. Retrieved from http://www.jointcommission.org/ assets/1/18/SEA_40.PDF

Martin, K. (2005). *The Omaha System: A key to practice, documentation, and information management* (reprinted 2nd ed.). Omaha, NE: Health Connections Press. Retrieved from http://omahasystem.org/

Martin, K., & Scheet, N. (1992). *The Omaha System: Applications for community health nursing.* Philadelphia: Saunders.

Merriam-Webster's Online Dictionary (11th ed.). (2011). Springfield, MA: Merriam-Webster.

Moorhead, S., Johnson, M., Maas, M., & Swanson, E. (2007). *Nursing outcomes classification* (NOC). St. Louis, MO: Mosby Elsevier.

Muller-Staub, M., Lavin, M., Needham, I., & van Achterberg, T. (2006). Nursing diagnoses, interventions and outcomes—application and impact on nursing practice: Systematic review. *Journal of Advanced Nursing, 56*(5), 514–531.

NANDA International. http://www.nanda.org/

National Association of Clinical Nurse Specialists (NACNS). (2009). *Core practice doctorate clinical nurse specialist competencies.* Retrieved from http://www.nacns.org/docs/CorePracticeDoctorate.pdf

National CNS Competency Task Force. (2010). *Clinical nurse specialist core competencies.* Philadelphia: National Association of Clinical Nurse Specialists. Retrieved from http://www.aacn.org/WD/Certifications/Docs/corecnscompetencies-execsumm.pdf

National Organization of Nurse Practitioner Faculties. (2006). *Domains and core competencies of nurse practitioner practice.* Washington, DC: Author. Retrieved from http://www.pncb.org/ptistore/resource/content/about/DomainsandCoreComps2006.pdf

The Omaha System: Solving the clinical data-information puzzle. http://www.omahasystem.org/

Peterson, C. (Ed.). (2011). *Perioperative nursing data set* (3rd ed.). Denver, CO: AORN, Inc.

Public Health Functions Steering Committee. (1994). 10 essential public health services. *Public Health in America.* Washington, DC: U.S. Public Health Services. Retrieved from http://www.cdc.gov/nphpsp/essentialServices.html

Rakel, R. (2011). Diagnosis. In *Encyclopedia Britannica.* Retrieved from http://www.britannica.com/EBchecked/topic/161063/diagnosis

Rivera, J., & Parris, K. (2002). Use of nursing diagnoses and interventions in public health nursing practice. *Nursing Diagnosis, 13*(1), 15–23.

Ruch, P., Gobeill, J., Lovis, C., Geissbühler, A. (2008). Automatic medical encoding with SNOMED categories. *BMC Medical Informatics and Decision Making. 8*(Suppl 1), S6. doi:10.1186/1472-6947-8-S1-S6

Rutherford, M. (2008). Standardized nursing language: What does it mean for nursing practice? *OJIN: Online Journal of Issues in Nursing, 13*(1). doi:10.3912/OJIN.Vol13No01PPT05

Saba, V. (2006). *Clinical care classification (CCC) system manual: A guide to nursing documentation.* New York, NY: Springer Publishing Company.

Satterfield, D., Murphy, D., Essien, J., Hosey, G., Stankus, M., Hoffman, P., Beartusk, K., Mitchell, P., & Alfaro-Correa, A. (2004). Using the essential public health services as strategic leverage to strengthen the public health response to diabetes. *Public Health Reports, 119*, 311–321.

Smith, K., & Bazini-Barakat, N. (2003). A public health nursing practice model: Melding public health principles with the nursing process. *Public Health Nursing, 20*(1), 42–48.

Stedman's Medical Dictionary (28th ed.). (2006). Baltimore, MD: Lippincott Williams & Wilkins.

Westra, B. (2005). *National health information infrastructure (NHII) and nursing: Implementing the Omaha system in community-based practice.* CareFacts Information Systems. Retrieved from http://www.himss.org/content/files/ImplementationNursingTerminologyCommunity.pdf

Wisc-Online Nursing vs. Medical Diagnosis: http://www.wisc-online.com

World Health Organization (WHO). (2007). *WHO international statistical classification of diseases and health-related problems* (10th revision). Retrieved from http://apps.who.int/classifications/apps/icd/icd10online/

World Health Organization (WHO). (2011). International Classification of Functioning, Disability and Health (ICF). Retrieved from http://www.who.int/classifications/icf/en/

Zielstorff, R. (1998). Characteristics of a good nursing nomenclature from an informatics perspective. *OJIN: Online Journal of Issues in Nursing, 3*(2). Retrieved from http://nursingworld.org/MainMenuCategories/ANAMarketplace/ANAPeriodicals/OJIN/TableofContents/Vol31998/No2Sept1998/CharacteristicsofNomenclaturefromInformaticsPerspective.aspx

CHAPTER 6

Standard 3. Outcomes Identification

Margaret G. Williams, PhD, RN, CNE, and
Kathleen M. White, PhD, RN, NEA-BC, FAAN

***Standard 3. Outcomes Identification.* The registered nurse identifies expected outcomes for a plan individualized to the healthcare consumer or the situation.**

Definition and Explanation of the Standard

The nursing community has defined an *outcome* as an individual's, family's, or community's state, behavior, or perception that can be measured along a continuum and is responsive to nursing interventions (University of Iowa, 2012). Discussions in today's healthcare environment expand that definition and identify the terms *outcome, expected outcome, desired outcome, goal,* and *objective* as interchangeable terms to describe a desired change in the healthcare consumer's health status or functioning. The nurse, using clinical knowledge and experience, determines outcomes in collaboration with the healthcare team and the healthcare consumer to provide individualized care and to delineate what is to be accomplished and when. This determination promotes the healthcare consumer's involvement in the care and enables measurement of the effectiveness of the plan.

Much as diagnoses are identified and prioritized from assessment data, outcomes identification refers to the formulation of specific, measurable, achievable, realistic, and time-framed (SMART) outcomes:

- *Specific:* The outcome must be clearly defined and understandable to all team members.

- *Measureable:* The team must be able to determine if the outcome is attainable and what improvement or movement must be accomplished (increase, decrease, size, and number).

- *Achievable:* All team members determine what the outcome should be.

- *Realistic:* The team agrees that the outcomes can be achieved with the current clinical condition and resources available.

- *Time-framed:* The team identifies the time needed to achieve the outcome.

Those outcomes are the statement of the healthcare consumer's status or progress that would demonstrate reduction, resolution, or prevention of a problem that was identified in the assessment and diagnosis steps of the nursing process, and they serve as criteria to evaluate the plan of care. Examples of SMART outcome statements are as follows:

- The healthcare consumer's temperature will decrease to normal or to baseline within four hours after administration of antipyretic medication.

- The healthcare consumer will reduce smoking to less than one pack per day within one month following daily administration of "the patch."

The outcomes identified in the plan may be either short-term or long-term. *Short-term* outcomes are those that can be achieved fairly quickly, within hours or days; that show progress toward resolution of a problem; and that are often a stepping stone toward reaching a long-term goal. A *long-term goal* often requires weeks or months to be achieved and usually reflects resolution or prevention of a problem.

In the past, healthcare outcomes that were determined to be nursing sensitive were those that were influenced by and improved by a greater quantity or quality of nursing care. In 1994, the American Nurses Association (ANA) launched the Patient Safety and Quality Initiative that funded a series of pilot studies to evaluate links between nurse staffing and quality of care (ANA, 1995). Several quality indicators were identified from those pilots, and a final set of 10 nursing-sensitive indicators to use in evaluating patient-care quality was adopted (Gallagher & Rowell, 2003).

The ANA established the National Database of Nursing Quality Indicators® (NDNQI®) in 1998 with the goals of (1) providing acute care hospitals with comparative information on nursing indicators that could be used in quality improvement projects and (2) developing a database that could be used to examine the relationship between aspects of the nursing workforce and nursing-sensitive patient outcomes (Dunton, Gajewski, Klaus, & Pierson, 2007; Montalvo, 2007). Outcome measures in the database that hospitals are collecting and reporting include but are not limited to the following:

- Patient fall rate.

- Injury from fall rate.

- Hospital-acquired pressure ulcer rate.

- Psychiatric patient injury assault rate.

- Prevalence of pediatric IV infiltration.

- Completeness of the pain assessment cycle for pediatric patients.

- Restraint prevalence.

- Urinary catheter-associated urinary tract infection for intensive care unit (ICU) patients.

- Central line catheter-associated blood stream infection rate for ICU and high-risk nursery (HRN) patients.

- Ventilator-associated pneumonia for ICU and HRN patients.

ANA has collaborated with The Joint Commission to include NDNQI as a recognized reporting mechanism for nursing outcomes, and several NDNQI outcome indicators have been endorsed by the National Quality Forum (NQF) through its voluntary consensus measurement identification process.

The nurse is also involved in identifying outcomes to design plans for improvement in direct and indirect nursing work, such as with groups, communities, populations, organizations, and systems. Examples of those outcomes may include the healthcare needs of an at-risk vulnerable population in a community or insurance plan, identification and planning for human capital needs in an organization, educational needs of a department or facility, or program planning quality and safety improvement for an organization or system. Outcomes for this nursing work, beyond the healthcare consumer and family, must also be based on comprehensive assessment and diagnosis and on using the SMART framework for outcomes identification to serve as a basis for planning, implementation, and evaluation.

Although it is generally recognized that outcomes should be individualized to the healthcare consumer or group, the use of standardized outcomes is necessary for the evaluation of nursing interventions, documentation in electronic records, use in clinical information systems, development of nursing knowledge, and education of professional nurses. Various tools are available to help the nurse identify approved and standardized outcomes.

Structure, Process, and Outcomes Model

Historically, the model of quality evaluation in health care proposed by Donabedian (1966/2005) identified three dimensions that are still useful for outcomes identification in health care and can be used in both direct and indirect nursing. The three dimensions are structure, process, and outcomes. *Structure* refers to the setting where care is provided, including equipment, staff, and programs, and assesses if the right things are in place to provide or access health care or alleviate the issue. *Process* determines the effectiveness, appropriateness, efficiency, and competency of care provided and assesses if the right things are being done to provide or access health care or alleviate the issue. *Outcomes* refer to the end points of care and ask if the right things are happening because of the actions of the providers.

Nursing Outcomes Classification

Another tool is the Nursing Outcomes Classification (NOC) developed and maintained by the University of Iowa's College of Nursing. The NOC is a comprehensive, standardized classification of patient and client outcomes that are sensitive or responsive to the effects of nursing interventions (University of Iowa, 2012). The NOC has identified 385 outcomes that can be used with all populations, in all settings, and across the care continuum to follow patient outcomes throughout an illness episode or over an extended period of care. The NOC is complementary to the Nursing Intervention Classification (NIC) system and has been linked to North American Nursing Diagnosis Association International (NANDA-I) diagnoses, to Marjorie Gordon's functional patterns, to the Taxonomy of Nursing Practice, to Omaha System problems, to resident admission protocols (RAPs) used in nursing homes, and to the Center for Medicare and Medicaid Services' Outcome and Assessment Information Set (OASIS) used in home care. NOC is recognized by the ANA, is included in the Metathesaurus for a Unified Medical Language at the National Library of Medicine, and is listed in the Cumulative Index to Nursing and Allied Health Literature (CINAHL®) index.

NOC outcomes are grouped into seven domains: Functional Health, Physiologic Health, Psychosocial Health, Health Knowledge and Behavior,

Perceived Health, Family Health, and Community Health. Each outcome has a definition, a list of indicators that can be used to evaluate patient status in relation to the outcome, references used in the development of the outcome, and a five-point Likert scale to measure patient status. Examples of scales used with the outcomes are as follows: 1 = Extremely compromised to 5 = Not compromised and 1 = Never demonstrated to 5 = Consistently demonstrated (Moorhead, Johnson, Maas, & Swanson, 2008, p. ix).

For example, the healthcare consumer is diagnosed with activity intolerance related to report of exertional fatigue, dyspnea, and clinical measurement of increased abnormal heart rate in response to activity. The suggested NOC Labels could include Endurance, Energy Conservation, Activity Tolerance, or Self-Care: Activities of Daily Living (ADLs). For this example, the nurse chooses the NOC label of activity tolerance and writes two outcomes:

- The healthcare consumer will participates in one 20-minute prescribed physical activity with resulting appropriate increases (within normal limits for this healthcare consumer) in heart rate and breathing rate three times per week for one month.

- The healthcare consumer demonstrates increased activity tolerance as measured by decrease in exertional fatigue and dyspnea in response to activity.

Omaha System

A third tool that can assist the nurse with outcomes identification is the Omaha System (Martin, 2005), another comprehensive standardized taxonomy to document nursing work. The Omaha System consists of three relational components: a problem classification system, an intervention scheme, and a problem rating scale for outcomes (Omaha, 2012a). The problem rating scale for outcomes identifies and evaluates client progress throughout the period of service. It also uses a Likert-type scale to measure the range of severity of three concepts:

- *Knowledge*, what the client knows (no knowledge to superior knowledge);

- *Behavior*, what the client does (not appropriate behavior to consistently appropriate behavior); and

- *Status*, the number and severity of the client's signs and symptoms or predicament (extreme signs or symptoms to no signs or symptoms).

An example of the Omaha System involves a healthcare consumer who does not follow the recommended dosage schedule for his or her medication. The domain is Health-Related Behaviors, with an intervention scheme or plan to teach and counsel (Omaha System, 2012b). The target or outcome is to increase knowledge about medication—its purpose and side effects—and to use a pill organizer to increase adherence to the medication schedule.

Some Characteristics of Outcome Identification

The Standards of Professional Nursing Practice identify eight competencies for the registered nurse in outcomes identification. The registered nurse must identify those desired outcomes with the healthcare consumer, his or her family, and caregivers, which the RN does in collaboration with other healthcare providers. In the outpatient setting, the nurse can ask the patient, "What is your goal for this visit?" In the inpatient setting, "What are the goals you hope to accomplish before discharge?"

Each outcome should be tailored specifically to the person and should be culturally appropriate. A person's background, culture, beliefs, and other dimensions all influence the desired outcomes. Thus, a question to ask could be: "Does this outcome reflect your belief systems, and is it practical for your life?" The associated risks, costs, and benefits should be discussed as part of such decision-making about desired outcomes. The outcomes must be based on evidence and must be designed as SMART outcomes that are specific to the change needed or expected; are measurable; are attainable for the healthcare consumer, family, or caregiver; are realistic; and have a time frame identified.

The graduate-level prepared specialty nurse and the APRN have additional expectations to ensure the use of scientific evidence in developing outcomes for the plan of care and interventions and in incorporating measures of cost, satisfaction, and continuity in the plans. Finally, the providers are expected to participate in individual- and system-level identification of outcomes.

Application of the Standard in Practice

Education

The nursing process is an important part of basic nursing education. Nurse educators are responsible for identifying each step of the process, teaching that step, and then putting the process back together while showing the interrelationship of the steps. For example, outcome identification depends on a comprehensive assessment and appropriate diagnosis of the healthcare consumer's problems or issues. Many nursing education programs teach the use of the NANDA-I classification for nursing assessment and diagnosis. The NOC and NIC are valuable tools that link with the NANDA-I classification for identification of outcomes and interventions. Incorporating those recognized approaches is important to standardize and define the knowledge base for nursing curricula and practice. Nurse educators must ensure competency and use of the nursing standardized languages across the curriculum.

The current emphasis on evidence-based practice demands that graduates have the skills and mechanisms to measure the outcomes of nursing care. The overall goal of nursing education is to prepare critical thinkers and to facilitate clinical decision-making. The outcome identification step in the nursing process is critical to this student development. The critical thinking approach requires that students are able to define and predict outcomes and to evaluate the effectiveness of their plans of care. In addition, nursing instructors need to teach students that discussing outcomes of care, which have been mutually agreed upon by the healthcare consumer and other providers, is a good way to facilitate and organize communication about the plan of care and effectiveness of nursing treatments to other nurses and providers.

Teaching the SMART technique for designing outcomes is appropriate for many situations, settings, and curricular levels, thereby requiring nurse educators to use their judgment and expertise when it may not be a beneficial format. However, using SMART ensures that the student will consider each part of the outcome identification and development process as they negotiate with the healthcare consumer and as they individualize to the situation and their circumstances.

Administration

The role of nursing administration in collecting nursing outcomes is essential in health care today. By evaluating outcomes, nursing administrators can assess the effectiveness of plans of care, improve team performance, and determine the adequacy of staffing and skill mix levels. Additionally, nurse administrators need to use all types of outcomes data to organize nursing; to plan for and evaluate use of financial, human, equipment, and physical resources; to facilitate performance and quality improvement efforts; and to publicly report outcomes that reflect the quality of safe and effective care.

The American Nurses Credentialing Center's Magnet Recognition Program® recognizes healthcare organizations for quality patient care, nursing excellence, and innovation in nursing practice. The Magnet Model® organizes 14 Forces of Magnetism® into five model components that focus on measurement outcomes. The fifth model component, Empirical Quality Results, posits that good outcomes will follow good structure and processes. It requires that Magnet facilities categorize outcomes by clinical outcomes related to nursing, workforce outcomes, patient and consumer outcomes, and organizational outcomes. Many Magnet-designated organizations or those seeking designation are reporting their outcomes to the previously discussed NDNQI. Through this reporting, nurse administrators receive benchmarked unit-level reports on how well they are meeting certain outcomes.

Nurse administrators help develop computerized information systems that enable nurses and other providers to identify and document outcomes of care. The systems also enable nurses to evaluate the healthcare consumer's response to the care provided and progress toward attainment of the outcome. However, those computerized systems are often untapped sources of data about the effectiveness of care. Nursing leadership must advance the collection, analysis, and evaluation of outcomes of care so nurses can identify additional outcomes, examine the cost of providing nursing care, and promote the development of a reimbursement system for nursing services. However, until those nursing data systems link the outcome identification step in the nursing process with the implementation and evaluation steps, nursing care effectiveness will remain undocumented. Nurse administrators must ensure that the work of nursing is visible, and they need the data to communicate the nature of nursing to the organization, to the public, and to policy-makers.

Performance and Quality Improvement

Identifying outcomes is critical to performance and quality improvement initiatives going on in most healthcare organizations today. Tools that use standardized languages are available to compare outcomes for improvement. Several were discussed earlier, such as the NOC and Omaha systems. Those classification systems standardize the outcome identification language for analysis, comparison, and improvement. The newest use of such classification systems in quality improvement is public reporting and value-based purchasing.

Research

The outcome identification step in the nursing process is important for research into the effectiveness of nursing personnel and the influence of nursing on the healthcare consumer's progress. There is a critical need to demonstrate that nursing care makes a difference and to show the cause and effect of nursing practice, such as linking the identification of outcomes to the healthcare consumer's response to the nursing plan of care and interventions.

The ANA established the National Center for Nursing Quality® (NCNQ®) in 1998. The NCNQ advocates for nursing quality through quality measurement and research. It also promotes research, using the NDNQI, to explore the relationship between nurse staffing and outcomes of patient care. There is also a need for research to identify new outcome measures.

Conclusion

Standard 3 Outcomes Identification describes the expectation that the registered nurse identifies expected outcomes for a plan individualized to the healthcare consumer or the situation. This third step in the nursing process requires competence in defining culturally appropriate expected outcomes for the healthcare consumer. The healthcare consumer helps formulate expected outcomes that facilitate continuity of care. The ability to estimate the time to attain the expected outcomes is another competency for this standard.

Case Study

Scenario Based on Person with Congestive Heart Failure

A 65-year-old male was seen in the outpatient clinic in severe congestive heart failure (CHF). He was then transferred to the emergency room, admitted to a telemetry unit for EKG monitoring and therapy for two days, and then transferred to a medical unit. Both a dietician and a physical therapist were involved in his care. At discharge, he was sent home with scheduled appointments at an outpatient CHF clinic. Referrals were made for outpatient cardiac rehabilitation and home care visits.

(Nursing care delivery should be in the type of setting you are familiar with in your health system. Include pertinent sociocultural information based on cultural diversity or cultural norms for your area [e.g., rural or urban].)

Learning Objectives

A. Using the NOC book (Moorhead, et al., 2008), describe the appropriate outcomes for this patient during all the phases of care.

B. Visit the IHI site, and contrast the outcomes listed there with what you have seen in your nursing practice.

OUTCOMES BASED ON IHI RECOMMENDATIONS
See the IHI site: http://www.ihi.org/explore/CHF/Pages/default.aspx.

C. Personalize the care for this patient by tailoring the outcomes to reflect different cultural and religious beliefs.

D. Contrast the outcomes for this patient based on being hospitalized in (1) different parts of the country, (2) different hospitals in the same 60-mile radius, and (3) rural versus urban locations by visiting http://www.hospitalcompare.hhs.gov.

E. While applying the best practice tools found at http://consultgerirn.org/resources, practice using assessment tools that may relate to this patient.

F. Devise different outcomes based on your assessment findings. Tools to consider: Mental Status Assessment of Older Adults: The Mini-Cog and the Geriatric Depression Scale, Fulmer SPICES: An Overall Assessment Tool for Older Adults, the Katz Index in Activities of Daily Living, and Informal Caregivers of Older Adults at Home (http://consultgerirn.org/resources).

G. Visit the IHI site at http://www.ihi.org/explore/CHF/, and practice using the tools listed under Congestive Heart Failure to create outcomes.

H. Using the above scenario, build on the case study to create the following:

- *Outcomes based on RN competencies*
  Assessment of knowledge
  Assessment of current medical regime

- *Outcomes based on advanced practice*
  Advanced assessment skills
  Prescription of medications

- *Outcomes based on administration*
  Readmission rates
  Inpatient and outpatient satisfaction

- *Outcomes based on quality initiatives*
  Consider measurement strategies at the IHI's Transforming Care at the Bedside and the Robert Wood Johnson Foundation web sites at

http://www.ihi.org/offerings/Initiatives/PastStrategicInitiatives/
TCAB/Pages/Materials.aspx and http://www.rwjf.org/qualityequal-
ity/product.jsp?id=30051.

- *Whole-system measures, business case measures, design target measures*
  Fall rates, pressure-ulcer prevalence, deaths among hospital surgical inpatients, and number of codes per month

References and Other Sources

American Nurses Association (ANA). (1995). *Nursing's report card for acute care.* Washington, DC: American Nurses Publishing.

Donabedian, A. (1966/2005). Evaluating the quality of medical care. *The Millbank Quarterly 83*(4), 691–729. (Reprinted from *The Milbank Memorial Fund Quarterly 44*(3), 166–203.)

Dunton, N., Gajewski, B., Klaus, S., & Pierson, B. (2007). The relationship of nursing workforce characteristics to patient outcomes. *OJIN: The Online Journal of Issues in Nursing 12*(3), Manuscript 3. doi:10.3912/OJIN.Vol12No03Man03

Gallagher, R. M., & Rowell, P.A. (2003). Claiming the future of nursing through nursing-sensitive quality indicators. *Nursing Administration Quarterly 24*(4), 273–284.

Martin, K. (2005). *The Omaha System: A key to practice, documentation, and information management* (2nd ed.). Omaha, NE: Health Connections Press.

Montalvo, I. (2007). The National Database of Nursing Quality Indicators. *OJIN: The Online Journal of Issues in Nursing 12*(3), Manuscript 2. doi:10.3912/OJIN.Vol12No03Man02

Moorhead, S., Johnson, M., Maas, M. L., & Swanson, E. (Eds.). (2008). *Nursing Outcomes Classification (NOC)* (4th ed.). St. Louis, MO: Mosby Elsevier.

NANDA International. http://www.nanda.org/

Omaha System (2012a) Omaha System overview. Retrieved from http://www.omahasystem.org/overview.html

Omaha System. (2012b). Omaha System problem classification schemes. Retrieved from http://omahasystem.org/problemclassificationscheme .html

University of Iowa, College of Nursing, Center for Nursing Classification & Clinical Effectiveness. (2012). *CNC—Overview: Nursing Outcomes Classification (NOC)*. Retrieved from http://www.nursing.uiowa.edu/ cncce/nursing-outcomes-classification-overview

CHAPTER 7

Standard 4. Planning

Jennifer Matthews, PhD, RN, ACNS-BC, CNE, FAAN

Standard 4. Planning. **The registered nurse develops a plan that prescribes strategies and alternatives to attain expected outcomes.**

Definition and Explanation of the Standard

The development of the plan or the strategies of action prescribed by the professional registered nurse (RN) is a foundational obligation of responsibility and accountability to the patient (ANA, 2001, 2010). The plan is the recorded document of the nurse's planned or intended course of action to provide professional nursing care to the healthcare consumer to help achieve the outcomes identified in the third step of the nursing process. This planning and the record of it are requirements of the regulatory agencies overseeing the provision of care to every patient in an accredited facility. The documentation of the planning is often referred to as a care plan, or a plan of care.

Three elements precede the planning of strategies for interventions: assessment, diagnosis, and identification of outcomes (see previous chapters). Each of the preceding phases in the nursing process contributes in a unique way to the planning phase. If not approached accurately and systematically, the plan may not be individualized or appropriate, and it may not directly target interventions that will contribute to high-quality patient outcomes. In the definition of nursing, two elements support the planning phase of care (ANA, 2010, p. 9):

- Integration of assessment data with knowledge gained from an appreciation of the patient or the group.

- Application of scientific knowledge to the process of diagnosis and treatment through the use of judgment and critical thinking.

Planning is the cognitive integrative process that relies on the previous steps and is characterized in the standards as a prescription of strategies. A *strategy* is an approach—a broader view—whereas a *tactic* is one specific action—an intervention or action for treatment. Planning is the keystone that unifies the initial interface between the nurse and the patient whereby they achieve the expected short-term or long-term outcomes of care. The planning phase is the critical cognitive aspect that *prescribes* the approach that comprises a set of interventions or treatments; it establishes the blueprint or is the "game-plan." To establish this plan, the nurse must critically think through an array of nursing approaches or interventions by considering, judging, accepting or rejecting, prioritizing, selecting, and organizing the interventions specific to the patient at that time.

This reasoning process is intangible and is based on the nurse's personal levels of knowledge, experience, and intuition, as well as the ability to execute psychomotor and psychosocial interventions, either alone or along with a multiskilled team. Inherent in this reasoning is the nurse's *anticipation* or *projection* of the effect of the interventions on the patient's condition—a focus on the outcomes. As a patient's condition changes, new assessment data inform the nurse to revise the planning and strategy selection for interventions that will meet the new needs. The plan and planning can be in constant change as priorities emerge.

The documentation of the planning phase relies on the standardized nursing terminologies and languages, such as those of the Nursing Outcomes Classification (NOC) and Nursing Interventions Classification (NIC) (University of Iowa, 2011). Those taxonomies are readily available and are part of content material in general fundamentals textbooks and courses (Craven & Hirnle, 2007). The plan is documented in the patient's permanent record to inform the interprofessional team members, including the patient, about the plan of action.

The complexity of this phase must be emphasized. In this phase, streams of factors intersect to create a unique plan to protect, promote, and optimize the health and abilities of an individual. The factors in planning are nurse-related, patient-based, resource-based, evidence-based, and environmental. Care planning is not static, but dynamic. Change occurs as the nurse matures along the novice-to-expert continuum of clinical practice (Benner, 1984), and the patient's status fluctuates acutely or imperceptibly along the wellness–illness continuum. The nurse's ability to create individualized planning improves as maturity

- Broadens the nurse's perception and insight in anticipating potential events.

- Tempers the nurse's judgment in weighing alternatives and options for optimal efficiency and effectiveness

- Improves the nurse's intuition about the time reality in executing the intervention.

Beyond physiologic changes, characteristics of the patient that affect the plan are level of ability; engagement, motivation, and despair; communication literacy; and support from significant others. Intersecting those dynamic continuums are resource factors that may affect the delivery of care designed within the care plan, such as the skill mix of assistive personnel, available supplies and equipment, availability of clinical experts, and unit support structure. The environment of care factors is the geographic design of the nursing unit, the levels of noise, the lighting, the available technology, and others. There is a continual state of inquiry in healthcare practice and delivery; knowledge is continuously being challenged. The nurse is the knowledge resource at the bedside and must translate evidence-proven research to practice the best in the art and science of nursing. The nurse must learn and renew knowledge through lifelong learning in planning and delivering nursing care.

As the nurse gains clinical practice experience, the nurse is better able to sort and filter information rapidly and more precisely. This information may be from the nurse's assessment of the patient or from assessments by clinical colleagues, which are communicated in the shift report through an SBAR (situation, background, assessment, recommendation report), in medical record documentation, or from the patient and family. In the past, the strategy for selecting interventions to achieve the expected outcome regularly relied on the nurse's memory and experience with interventions and might have included interventions that were not proven effective in care delivery. Currently, reliance on accepted evidence-based practices, use of collaboratively created critical pathways, incorporation of care taxonomies, and use of available computer technology allow more options for the nurse to select from, thus resulting in increased varieties of interventions (Clancy, Delaney, Morrison, & Gunn, 2006).

The norm today is for use of care plans that are the outcomes of collaborative efforts by interprofessional teams, and the planning enhances continuity of care. As each nurse accepts the responsibility for a patient's care, either in a shift bedside report or at a point of entry into the healthcare system, the tandem responsibility is to plan, communicate, and record the individualized care strategies. This endeavor is accomplished by beginning an assessment and moving the process forward to the planning phase. The nurse can review the patient's previous plan and accept or confirm it. Or the nurse can modify the plan so that it remains unique and individualized for the patient at this time. The nurse must actively determine—that is, plan—the strategies and then the interventions necessary to achieve the expected outcomes for the individual. The nurse individualizes the projected outcomes for the patient.

The National Council of State Boards of Nursing (NCSBN), which develops and administers the national licensure examination (NCLEX), tests the integration of nursing material. Skill in planning is essential because as many as 22% of NCLEX test items focus on client management of care (NCSBN, 2009, p. 4). The planning standard of practice (ANA, 2010) provides suggestions for the strategies to address each of the identified diagnoses or issues:

- Promote and restore health.

- Prevent illness, injury, and disease.

- Alleviate suffering.

- Provide supportive care for the individual who is dying.

- Execute the orders of a licensed provider.

The scope of practice for the RN in all states and territories depends on specialized education, planning and judgment, and skills based on knowledge and application of principles. Licensed practical (vocational) nurses are not allowed to plan the care of a patient in the acute care setting; they are allowed to perform technical skills and implement the plan under the direction of an RN.

The graduate-level prepared specialty nurses or advanced practice registered nurses (APRNs) function at greater levels of complexity of planning. Their expertise in specialty knowledge and comprehensive practice permits insight and planning for broader strategies in managing multifaceted, complex individuals or populations. In this role, the graduate-level prepared specialty nurse may initiate and lead the plan design or the planning for clinical integration that meets the needs of individuals or populations. APRNs establish the planning strategies that may include nursing care interventions or medical therapies that are executed by licensed or unlicensed personnel. The planning encompasses continuous improvement of systems that support the planning process itself.

Application of the Standard in Practice

Education

For nursing students, the nurse educators design instructional content that aligns with the national standards of educational practice, as well as the national standards of nursing practice (ANA, 2010; CCNE, 2009; NLNAC, 2008). Those standards include planning as part of the nursing process. Nursing students create instructional care plans that are learning tools to aid them in learning the process of care planning while using critical thinking and evidence. The faculty provides guidance and feedback to the student about each aspect of the plan and care. Through the repetitive exercise in developing the instructional care plans, a progression occurs that allows the novice RN to enter practice with a basic skill set to plan and manage the care of individual patients.

Administration

Nurse administrators use the nursing process as they determine (assess) the scope of an issue, diagnose or label the situation, determine the ideal outcomes, and then *plan* the strategies to achieve the outcomes. Those business plans are formulated for a wide range of issues that directly affect nurses and patient care, for example, how to secure more RN positions, how to achieve greater productivity, how to manage the resources that affect direct patient care, or how to create a healing environment for the patient. The nurse administrator must ensure that the process of planning is part of the position description for every nurse. Many position descriptions use the nursing process as the format for clinical responsibility and performance appraisal.

Performance and Quality Improvement

In 1996, ANA took bold steps to advance the centrality of nurses in the care of patients with the launching of the Magnet Recognition Program® and the

National Database for Nursing Quality Indicators®. The overwhelming and undisputed outcomes of those two programs have been the dramatic focus on quality nursing care and improved patient care outcomes. The critical factors in achieving high benchmark levels of nursing care are the planning and the implementation of the care, which depend on nursing judgment and planning. Organizations involved in analyzing healthcare initiatives, such as the Institute of Medicine (IOM), The Joint Commission (TJC), and the Institute for Healthcare Improvement (IHI), rely on the outcomes of nursing care for the measures they create to ensure safe and effective patient care. The outcomes can be measured as shorter lengths of stay in the hospitals, lower rates of readmission, lower infection rates while in the hospitals, or fewer falls by patients during hospitalization. The unit-level and hospital-wide outcomes occur because the nurses accountable for the care planned and selected the individual interventions; expert planning is quality care for quality improvement.

Research

Through Benner's seminal research work of *From Novice to Expert* (1984), the profession understands the progression of the nurse (or the learner) in managing and anticipating patient care. This progression is based in part on the accomplishment of skills but mostly on the cognitive development of the judgment and emotional maturity of the nurse. Judgment and maturity are dominant in *planning* the nursing care while using critical analysis and sorting the options to find the best solution for the patient's problem. This planning is an approach that sets the tone for the level and depth of caring and for the patient's participation in the healing and recovery journey to achieve the expected outcomes. The highest level of comprehensive planning is a holistic patient-centered approach.

Benner extended her research in 2010 and suggested that the assignments of written clinical instructional care plans should be fewer and well-tempered with other indicators of clinical performance. She states that, while in the learning setting, the educator should determine "how well students are able to set priorities . . . and that students should also be assessed on their skills of clinical reasoning and their ability to solve clinical puzzles" (Benner, Sutphen, Leonard, & Day, 2010, p. 221). Those recommendations need educational research and evaluation so that the profession can gain insight into how clinical reasoning, judgment, and decision-making develop, as well as the factors that affect such decisions.

Conclusion

Standard 4 Planning describes the expectation that the RN develops a plan that prescribes strategies and alternatives to achieve expected outcomes. This fourth step in the nursing process requires competence in establishing priorities and strategies with the healthcare consumer that address each of the identified diagnoses or issues. Consideration of the economic impact on the healthcare consumer and current scientific evidence, trends, and research inform the planning effort.

Case Study with Discussion Topics

C is a 76-year-old widower who was admitted to the hospital for stabilization of his medical problems. He lives alone; his wife died 2 years ago and had cared for him meticulously. In effect, she was his case manager. C is diagnosed with systolic heart failure.

Assessment: Step 1 of the nursing process

The assessment data that reveal the clinical manifestations of his medical condition are these:

- Myocardial infarction (MI) 10 years ago.

- Cardiac surgery (CABG) 9 years ago.

- Weight 120 kg (264 lbs) (up from a typical 114 kg).

- Heart rate—104, occasionally irregular.

- BP—165/95 mmHg.

- Ejection fraction (EF) 40%.

- Shortness of breath; rate at 28 breaths per minute auscultation reveals rales and crackles in the base region of the lung

- Oxygen saturation at 90

- Bilateral lower extremity—2+ – 3+ pitting edem

- A1C (HbA_1C) is 9.8

- B-type natiuretic peptide (BNP)—8,559 *pg.*

C has three nursing diagnoses:

- Decreased cardiac output related to reduced myocardial perfusion as related to damaged cardiac muscle (MI and EF).

- Ineffective ventilation or breathing pattern as related to inability to maintain adequate rate and depth of respirations as evidenced by the vital signs and low O_2 saturation.

- Fluid volume excess related to excess fluid retention or excess sodium intake or retention as evidence by lower extremity edema and pulmonary congestion.

Three primary nursing goals are these:

- Improve the functioning of the cardiac muscle.

- Improve the patient ventilatory effort leading to improved oxygenation.

- Reduce the fluid volume available for third spacing into the lungs and interstitial tissues.

Planning: Step 4 of the nursing process. See the table below, Ventilatory Functions of Case Study Subject C, and the discussion.

Interventions and implementation: Step 5 of the nursing process.

Outcomes evaluation: Step 6 of the nursing process.

The desired expected outcomes are for C to have optimal function for his activities of daily living through the following:

- Adequate cardiac output (ejection fraction) for tissue perfusion.

- Efficient ventilatory function for improved oxygenation of all tissues.

- Regulated fluid balance, with sodium intake restriction, so that fluid intake approximates the fluid output or loss.

Planning: Step 4 of the nursing process

Planning is the strategic approach that brings the objective data—the individualism of the patient—into combination with the clinician's expertise to formulate the plan of action, design the game plan, and select the interventions or tactics that will achieve the expected outcomes. This keystone step unites the first three steps and links them to the expected outcomes. The characteristics and experience of the nurse will be a significant influence on the interventions selected.

For example, the following table addresses the ventilatory functions of this patient.

Ventilatory Functions of Case Study Subject C

	Novice Nurse	Experienced Nurse	Expert Nurse
Planning (step 4)	Task-oriented planning	Organized planning that includes teaching	Holistic planning
Interventions (step 5)	Measure and record vital signs. Listen to lungs after report. Weigh C each morning. Administer and record medications. Tell patient to limit salt intake.	Assess, monitor, and trend the vital signs, weight, and lab parameters throughout the shift. Coach the patient about effects of typical medications used for heart failure. Provide literature on salt-restricted diets. Encourage C to be out of bed, and inform RN of shortness of breath (SOB) or respiratory difficulties.	Determine C's baseline knowledge of his condition, heart failure, and diabetes. Determine C's living situation: cultural values surrounding food, ability to prepare meals, and financial ability to purchase foods that avoid sodium and are compatible with a diabetic menu. Determine C's emotional adjustment to loss of wife. Engage planning with the multidisciplinary team members.
Outcomes (step 6)	Vital signs are recorded. Lung sounds are described. Weight is recorded. Medications are administered, and the effects may be noted in the amount of fluid output, the improvement of lung sounds, the amount of weight loss, and the reduction in lower extremity edema. C knows he is not to add salt to his food.	The nurse monitors and seeks positive changes in the vital signs, weight loss, and improvement in labs that signify the stress of heart failure. The patient can repeat the effects of his medication. The patient reads the instructions on salt-restricted diets. The patient is out of bed and monitors self for respiratory changes.	The nurse discovers that the patient knows little to nothing about his medical conditions. His wife cared for him, and he let her do everything. The nurse discovers that the patient and his culture put great emphasis on "family" and eating together. He eats alone and only what is easy for him to heat or fix. Neighbors send food to him every couple of days. The patient is situationally depressed, and this is now close to clinical depression. He is not adjusting well to the loss of his wife, and he has little interest in events. The nurse determines he needs and can benefit from the expertise of a social worker, dietitian, physical therapist, and heart failure case manager.

Discussion Topics

1. Continue outlining the table for the types of interventions that the novice nurse, the experienced nurse, and the expert nurse would select to address the cardiac improvement and the fluid volume balance.

2. If you were the novice nurse, what approach should an experienced nurse use with you to help you learn and gain the experience to move to the beginner or intermediate phase?

3. Reflect on how you have been taught the nursing process and planning. What learning assignment would aid you in comprehending the nursing process?

4. Think about a patient you have cared for and have written a care plan about. Do you believe you could improve it? How would it be different now from how it was when you created it?

References and Other Sources

Alfaro-LeFevre, R. (2010). *Applying nursing process: A tool for critical thinking* (7th ed.). Philadelphia, PA: Wolters Kluwer Health: Lippincott Williams & Wilkins.

American Nurses Association (ANA). (2001). *Code of Ethics for Nurses with interpretive statements.* Washington, DC: American Nurses Publishing.

American Nurses Association (ANA). (2010). *Nursing's social policy statement: The essence of the profession.* Silver Spring, MD: Nursesbooks. org.

American Nurses Association (ANA). (2011). *National Database for Nursing Quality Indicators®.* Retrieved from https://www.nursingquality.org/

American Nurses Credentialing Center (ANCC). (2011). *ANCC Magnet Recognition Program.* Retrieved from http://www.nursecredentialing.org/ Magnet.aspx

Benner, P. (1984). *From novice to expert.* Menlo Park, CA: Addison Wesley.

Benner, P., Sutphen, M., Leonard, V., & Day, L. (2010). *Educating nurses: A call for radical transformation.* San Francisco, CA: Jossey-Bass.

The Essential Guide to Nursing Practice

Clancy, T. R., Delaney, C. W., Morrison, B., & Gunn, J. K. (2006). The benefits of standardized nursing languages in complex adaptive systems such as hospitals. *Journal of Nursing Administration, 36*(9), 426–434.

Commission on Collegiate Nursing Education (CCNE). (2009). *Standards for accreditation of baccalaureate and graduate degree nursing programs.* Washington, DC: Author.

Craven, R. F., & Hirnle, C. J. (2007). *Fundamentals of nursing: Human health and function* (5th ed.). Philadelphia, PA: Lippincott Williams & Wilkins.

Institute of Medicine. (2011). *The future of nursing: Leading change, advancing health.* Washington, DC: National Academies Press.

NANDA-I – North American Nursing Diagnosis Association—International. (2011). Retrieved from http://www.nanda.org/

National Council of State Boards of Nursing (NCSBN). (2009). 2010 NCLEX-RN® test plan: National council licensure examination for registered nurses. Retrieved from https://www.ncsbn.org/2010_NCLEX_RN_TestPlan.pdf

National League for Nursing Accrediting Commission (NLNAC). (2008). *Standards and criteria for baccalaureate programs.* Retrieved from http://www.nlnac.org/manuals/SC2008.htm

University of Iowa, College of Nursing. (2011). Center for Nursing Classification and Clinical Effectiveness. Retrieved from http://www.nursing.uiowa.edu/center-for-nursing-classification-and-clinical-effectiveness

CHAPTER 8
Standard 5. Implementation

Beth Martin, MSN, RN, CCNS, ACNP-BC, ACHPN

Standard 5. Implementation. **The registered nurse implements the identified plan.**

> *Standard 5A. Coordination of Care.* **The registered nurse coordinates care delivery.**
>
> *Standard 5B. Health Teaching and Health Promotion.* **The registered nurse employs strategies to promote health and a safe environment.**
>
> *Standard 5C. Consultation.* **The graduate-level prepared specialty nurse or advanced practice registered nurse provides consultation to influence the identified plan, enhance the abilities of others, and effect change.**
>
> *Standard 5D. Prescriptive Authority and Treatment.* **The advanced practice registered nurse uses prescriptive authority, procedures, referrals, treatments, and therapies in accordance with state and federal laws and regulations.**

Definition and Explanation of the Standard

The plan of care developed in the previous three standards is actualized through the implementation standard. In this phase of the nursing process, nurses continue to use clinical judgment and critical thinking to prepare themselves, the healthcare consumer, and the environment for action. Planned interventions are carried out to help the client achieve identified outcomes.

Implementation requires nurses to combine thinking and doing, as well as feeling, sensing, and valuing. Nurses select and implement interventions that promote client goal achievement. The interventions may be delegated, independent, or interdependent actions. Independent nursing actions are autonomous and occur when the nurse conducts assessments and interventions for the purpose of promoting health and healing. The focus is on the client's response to actual or potential health problems.

Nurses also implement delegated interventions, such as those that are required standard or protocol or are ordered by other providers such as physicians or nurse practitioners. Nurses carry out those delegated functions when their knowledge, experience, and judgment confirm that the order is appropriate and safe for the client. (Koularatis, 2004). In interdependent practice, nurses collaborate with other disciplines to jointly identify and implement specialized interventions.

Implementation involves direct client care as well as indirect care. Direct care includes the use of cognitive skills (critical thinking, reflection, clinical judgment, creativity, etc.); interpersonal skills (caring, communication, comforting, advocacy, counseling, etc.); and technical or psychomotor skills (lifting, giving injections, repositioning, etc.). Indirect care interventions are those carried out away from the client, such as managing the environment or consulting with a specialist.

Implementation may involve delegation of actions to other nurses or healthcare workers. The nurse is accountable for the quality of care provided directly, indirectly, or through delegation. Professional and legal standards for delegation must be followed. Nurse administrators, educators, and others in graduate-level specialty prepared roles use implementation as they carry out the plans and goals developed in prior steps of the process.

It is during implementation of the plan that nurses *demonstrate* the art and science of nursing practice. The science of nursing is based on principles of the biological, physical, behavioral, and social sciences. Nurses integrate evidence with the practice-generated data, the clinical expertise, and the values and preferences of their clients to achieve goals. New knowledge is constantly used to inform practice and promote effective interventions (ANA, 2010a).

The art of nursing is based on caring and respect for human dignity. Caring is central to nursing practice and is demonstrated in the personal relationship that the nurse enters into with the client (ANA 2010b, p. 23). In a holistic framework for implementation, the nurse establishes an active partnership with the client; performs care with purposeful, focused intention; and recognizes the importance of the client's humanness. The presence of the caring nurse is, in and of itself, a therapeutic intervention (Potter & Frisch, 2009).

Nurses are responsible and accountable for maintaining and demonstrating their competence when implementing the plan of care. Knowledge, skills, abilities, and judgment, all of which are based on established science and current practice expectations, must be integrated in the nurse's actions (AACN, 2008). Nurses must assess their own competence and seek consultation or collaboration from appropriate sources if the client's needs are beyond their capabilities (ANA, 2001).

Implementation of interventions will generate patient responses and, therefore, inherently involve ongoing assessment and evaluation. Assessment information discovered during implementation informs evaluation and provides feedback on all other steps of the nursing process (ANA, 2010b). Nurses critically reflect during and after the implementation of interventions; the plan is constantly reassessed and modified to promote goal achievement.

A wealth of work has been done to identify and classify nursing interventions. The Center for Nursing Classification and Clinical Effectiveness at the University of Iowa's College of Nursing was established in 1995 to facilitate the ongoing research of the Nursing Interventions Classification (NIC). NIC is a comprehensive, research-based, standardized classification of interventions that nurses perform. The classification includes the interventions that nurses do on behalf of patients, both independent and collaborative interventions, both direct and indirect care.

The following examples demonstrate the broad range of interventions nurses implement, including strategies to promote health and a safe environment (Standard 5B), physiological (e.g., Acid–Base Management), psychosocial (e.g., Anxiety Reduction), illness treatment (e.g., Hyperglycemia Management), illness prevention (e.g., Fall Prevention), and health promotion (e.g., Exercise Promotion). Those interventions are all included in NIC. Most of the interventions are for use with individuals, but many are for use with families (e.g., Family Integrity Promotion) and some are for use with entire communities (e.g., Environmental Management—Community).

Indirect care interventions (e.g., Supply Management) are also included. The classification is continually updated with an ongoing process for feedback and review (University of Iowa, n.d.). The nurse uses knowledge and critical thinking to select and prioritize individualized interventions. Effective planning and implementation of appropriate interventions enhance client outcomes.

In practice, nurses demonstrate the implementation competencies when providing interventions in partnership with the healthcare consumer. Nurses demonstrate a caring approach in all interventions. Nurses introduce themselves and inform clients of the nurse's role in their care. They discuss the planned interventions and ensure client understanding. Clients are familiarized with their environment, and the purpose of any equipment used in their care is explained. Caring is demonstrated when nurses ensure client comfort (physical, emotional, and spiritual), privacy, and dignity while implementing interventions. Interventions are not initiated without the healthcare consumer or surrogate decision-maker's knowledge and consent. Great consideration is given to the healthcare consumer's readiness and ability to participate.

Interventions are implemented in a manner that respects client diversity. A nurse uses nonverbal communication and an interpreter when working with a client whose language he or she does not speak. He or she uses touch respectfully and cautiously for a client who is anxious or fearful. Religious and cultural beliefs regarding health care are honored in the nurse's approach to implementation of interventions.

Nurses use critical thinking skills as they determine *how* to implement interventions. All clients are individuals with diverse needs. A client's age, educational level, functional ability, and cultural and spiritual beliefs are but a few examples of individual characteristics that a nurse will consider when providing care. For example, an intervention such as skin care will be approached differently for an infant than for an older adult. How a client is taught to self-administer medications will vary according to a client's communication, language, and learning style preferences. Nurses use evidence-based interventions that are specific to a client's diagnosis; they also use the best evidence available to guide care delivery.

Nurses become expert at determining when interventions need to be modified on the basis of diverse client needs. Nurses apply a holistic framework to their thinking and recognize that effective implementation of interventions requires attention to the human dimensions of their clients. Wound care may go more smoothly when a loving parent holds the young child being cared for on his or her lap during the procedure. A client's anxiety may be eased when the spouse walks next to her or him on the ride to the operating room. Respect for privacy and confidentiality may promote honest dialogue when counseling a teenager. Multiple nursing theories and frameworks describe the personal relationships between client and nurse as well as caring processes and specific techniques (ANA, 2010a).

Recommendations from multiple organizations provide the nurse with guidance for timeliness and safety regarding implementation practices. High-risk activities such as medication administration are also guided by regulatory standards, as well as the nurse's knowledge, skills, and abilities. For example, The Joint Commission National Patient Safety Goals recommends that the nurse should use two ways to identify patients correctly. Before administering medication, the nurse will properly identify the patient. The nurse may ask the adult hospitalized client to state his or her name and date of birth and then may verify this information against the client's medical record and name band. This method of implementing correct identification of the client would vary in a nonverbal or cognitively impaired client (The Joint Commission, 2011).

Nurses may use technology to implement and enhance nursing practice, to coordinate client care, and to maximize client independence. Technology may be used in direct client care to collect physiologic data (cardiac monitors) or to provide support for physiologic function (mechanical ventilators). Nursing care is provided in highly technological environments, such as emergency departments, operating rooms, and intensive care units. In addition to effectively using the technology to optimize client outcomes, nurses manage the interface between the client and the technology. The use of technology may be frightening or threatening for a client. Nurses implement interventions to ensure that client safety and dignity are respected.

In the midst of highly technological environments, nurses ensure that clients experience a healing, humane approach (AACN, 2008). Nurses use technology indirectly to provide interventions. Telephonic monitoring is just one example of how nurses implement interventions such as health teaching, monitor responses to interventions, and ensure that clients have access to healthcare resources. Nurses may use technology to coordinate the interprofessional team and "hand off" communication within the systems for the client and family.

Graduate-level prepared specialty nursing practice builds on the competencies of registered nurses (RNs). Advanced practice registered nurses (APRNs) demonstrate all competencies related to direct patient care. Additionally, they use broader resources to implement interventions. APRNs demonstrate greater depth and breadth of knowledge, more advanced skills, and increased role autonomy. The defining factor for all APRNs is that a significant component of the education and practice focuses on direct care of individuals (APRN CWG & the NCSB, 2008, p. 7). The graduate-level specialty prepared nurse may facilitate a change in the policies and procedures of a healthcare system to meet client needs. APRNs are often instrumental in developing and implementing evidence-based protocols to promote optimal outcomes. They also practice closely with the healthcare team to implement change if client outcomes are not being met.

APRNs in the acute care setting collaborate with the team to review and revise plans of care and implement advanced interventions such as bedside surgical procedures. For example, the APRN may insert invasive monitoring devices and place chest drainage tubes. In the outpatient setting, an APRN may be a client's primary care provider, thereby implementing and coordinating disease-specific management.

Tracy (2009) describes six characteristics of direct clinical care that is provided by APRNs:

- APRNs use a holistic perspective, taking into account the complexity of human life.

- APRNs consider the profound effects of illness and stress when selecting and implementing care interventions.

- APRNs are expert at forming therapeutic partnerships with clients and are aware of potential cultural influences on healthcare decisions.

- APRNs acquire specialized knowledge that allows them to generate and test alternate lines of reasoning and demonstrate expert clinical thinking and skillful performance.

- APRNs apply reflective practice approaches and use evidence to guide their practice.

- APRNs use diverse approaches to health and illness management, coordinating care among sites and providers.

Evidence for this framework exists, and it substantiates the confidence of the nursing profession and the public in the direct care provided by APRNs.

This standard is unique in that there are four supplementary standards. Standard 5A, Coordination of Care, and Standard 5B, Health Teaching and Health Promotion, relate the responsibility to coordinate delivery of care and to use strategies to promote health and a safe environment. Standard 5C, Consultation, and Standard 5D, Prescriptive Authority and Treatment, are additional responsibilities for graduate-level prepared specialty nurses or APRNs.

Standard 5A. Coordination of Care

The nurse coordinates care delivery by organizing the components of the plan of care, assisting the client to identify alternative care options, communicating with all involved parties during care transitions, advocating for the client, and documenting the care coordination. Nurses coordinate delivery of care, use of physical resources (supplies and equipment), delegation of nursing care, and care provided by other disciplines. For example, a client may have a planned set of interventions to promote heart health through diet and activity. The nurse coordinates the care for this client with the interprofessional team members and available resources to help the client achieve the goals.

Standard 5B. Health Teaching and Health Promotion

The nurse provides health teaching and health promotion using appropriate methods for each individual client and situation. The nurse may implement the appropriate teaching and may coordinate teaching and therapies provided by a dietitian or cardiac rehabilitation specialist. The nurse may use web-based or other electronic media resources if they are available and consistent with the client's learning preferences. The nurse's decision about how and when to implement teaching interventions is influenced by the client's health practices, socioeconomic status, and readiness to learn. The nurse provides information about intended and potential side effects of proposed therapies. Health teaching and promotion interventions are documented appropriately so that the healthcare team has ongoing access to information about the care provided to promote client safety and continuity of care.

Standard 5C. Consultation

Standard 5C describes consultation competencies specific to APRNs and graduate-level prepared specialty nurses. Those nurses are able to provide consultation in their areas of expertise. The consultation is based on their specialized knowledge, skills, and abilities, often making them the "go to" person when expert advice is needed. For example, nurse educators may consult with clinical nurses and nurse managers to develop continuing education classes on clinical and professional topics as identified by needs assessments, client outcomes, quality improvement initiatives, or employee satisfaction issues.

Standard 5D. Prescriptive Authority and Treatment

Standard 5D describes the prescriptive authority for APRNs. The role of an APRN includes the use and prescription of pharmacologic and nonpharmacologic interventions (APRN CWG & NCSB, 2008). APRNs prescribe evidence-based, individualized pharmacologic and nonpharmacologic interventions and therapies in accordance with state and federal laws and regulations. APRNs evaluate the effectiveness of the treatments and interventions that are prescribed. APRNs also provide information about the prescribed treatments and procedures, including intended and potential adverse effects, costs, alternative treatments, and procedures to the healthcare consumer. When allowed, APRNs prescribe medications for disease and symptom management. APRNs prescribe referrals to other providers such as medical specialists, therapists, and counselors. Complementary, alternative, and nonpharmacologic therapies are also incorporated into the array of interventions that may be prescribed.

Application of the Standard in Practice

Education

The nurse educator implements the plan for educating students following the assessment of student learning needs and on the basis of the course objectives and curricular learning outcomes. The nurse educator also coordinates the educational process and teaches care coordination to nursing students.

Creating and maintaining healthy, safe learning environments are critical components of the educator's role. This environment can be created through implementation of mutual respect, open and honest communication, and safe learning experiences. Nurse educators implement programs that enhance the communication and collaboration skills of the nursing staff members, who enhance implementation of quality care.

Administration

Nurse administrators build on the RN competencies to promote practice environments characterized by nursing foundations for quality of care, nurse manager ability, leadership and support, and collegial nurse–physician relations. Those characteristics are associated with better client outcomes (Aiken, 2008). Nurse administrators consider the staff holistically and implement interventions to create a healthy work environment on the basis of their assessments.

Nurse administrators adopt and adapt nursing care delivery models to guide nursing care and implement policies and procedures to hold staff members accountable for implementing evidence-based standards of care throughout the entire healthcare system. Evaluation and performance appraisal systems are implemented to ensure that nurses are held accountable to those standards. Coaching, mentoring, and educating are implemented for nurses to assist them to meet the performance standards. Shared governance systems are implemented to involve nurses in developing care delivery models, policies, and procedures. Nurses in advanced practice roles are supported by nursing leadership to evaluate their practice and are held accountable for advanced levels of care.

Research

The goal of evidence-based nursing practice is to implement the best possible evidence to provide quality health care that meets expected outcomes to resolve problems as designed in the plan of care for the patient. This implementation involves two levels of action:

- First, nurses must question and critically appraise the evidence for implementation of interventions used in nursing practice.

- Second, nurses must design and implement research to evaluate interventions in nursing. Research evaluating the implementation of physiological, psychosocial, and educational interventions will contribute to the advancement of nursing science and will improve the quality of health and health care

The improvement of health care in the United States is a national priority. The National Institute of Nursing Research (NINR) supports clinical, biological, and translational research in many areas, including interventions aimed at symptom management, disease prevention, chronic illness, patient-focused health programs, and innovative methods that optimize patient outcomes and that provide cost-effective patient-focused interventions. Nurse-led intervention research to evaluate the implementation of patient care strategies will provide the scientific evidence for future interventions to improve the health of the public.

Nurses need to be involved in comparative-effectiveness research that is designed to inform healthcare decisions by providing evidence on the effectiveness, benefits, and harms of different treatment options. The evidence is generated from research studies that compare drugs, medical devices, tests, surgeries, or ways to deliver health care. Researchers look at all of the available evidence about the benefits and harms of each choice for different groups of people from *existing* clinical trials, clinical studies, and other research, or researchers conduct studies that generate *new* evidence of effectiveness or comparative effectiveness of a test, treatment, procedure, or healthcare service (AHRQ, 2011).

Comparative effectiveness research (CER) compares the effectiveness of two or more healthcare interventions. By making direct comparisons between a particular technology or treatment and an established standard of care or other realistic comparator, CER assesses how well a healthcare treatment or intervention works under real-world conditions (Lewin Group, 2011).

Performance and Quality Improvement

Nurses collaborate with other healthcare providers and must be involved in projects to implement evidence-based interventions. One such process is the Model for Improvement, which is a tool for accelerating improvement (IHI, 2011). It is not meant to replace change models currently in use, but to accelerate improvement initiatives. There are several parts to the model:

- Form the team.

- Set the aim.

- Establish measures.

- Test the change. The Plan-Do-Study-Act (PDSA) cycle is used to test changes in real work settings. The PDSA cycle uses a small test of change by planning, trying, observing results, and acting on what is learned to quickly determine if the change is likely to be effective. The PDSA cycle is shorthand for testing a change in the real work setting. This is the scientific method adapted for action-oriented learning.

- Implement the change. After testing a change on a small scale, learning from each test, and refining the change through several PDSA cycles, the team may implement the change on a broader scale, for example, for an entire pilot population or on an entire unit.

- Spread the change.

Conclusion

Standard 5 Implementation describes the expectation that the RN implements the identified plan, coordinates care delivery, and uses strategies to promote health and a safe environment. Consultation and prescriptive authority and treatment are graduate-level activities. This fifth step in the nursing process requires competence in using evidence-based interventions and treatments; in collaborating with healthcare providers to implement and integrate the plan; and in partnering with the person, family, and others to implement the plan in a safe, realistic, and timely manner.

Case Study with Discussion Topics

Case Study

John Ramirez underwent a colectomy for removal of a colon mass yesterday. The pathology report is pending; there is concern that the patient has colon cancer. He is a 67-year-old retired teacher. The nurse prepares herself to care for Mr. Ramirez by receiving a report from the off-going shift and reviewing the patient's medical record and plan of care. She learns that Mr. Ramirez did not sleep well and received pain medication three times on the previous 12-hour shift. She reviews the medical orders and the relevant surgical standards of care and protocols.

She self-assesses her knowledge and abilities related to this patient's care, including consideration of cultural sensitivities for care of Hispanic people. She recognizes that a new protocol for venous thromboembolism (VTE) prevention has been initiated. Because she is unfamiliar with the new protocol, she collaborates with the Clinical Nurse Specialist (CNS) on her unit. The CNS shares the evidence used to develop this protocol and explains the rationale for the practice change. Together they review the protocol and determine the appropriate interventions for Mr. Ramirez.

The goals for Mr. Ramirez include adequate pain management, increased mobility, and prevention of complications. She considers the goals to be achieved and uses critical thinking to select independent nursing interventions. She uses critical thinking skills to prioritize the interventions planned for Mr. Ramirez today. The nurse knows that his pain will need to be well controlled in order for him to participate in the planned care and to move toward goal achievement. The nurse is now ready to implement the plan of care.

The nurse approaches Mr. Ramirez and introduces herself. She begins her daily assessment and observes nonverbal signs of pain. Mr. Ramirez rates his pain 6 on a 1 to 10 scale. He reports that the pain medication brings the pain score to an acceptable level but wears off quickly. The nurse completes a physical assessment, with focused consideration of the patient's recent surgery.

His abdomen is not distended, but it is quite tender to light palpation. She repositions Mr. Ramirez and ensures that his nasogastric tube is draining correctly. She asks Mr. Ramirez about his priority needs or concerns today. He acknowledges that his pain needs to be better controlled, and he is anxious about the possibility of cancer. She asks about his support system and whether he expects any visitors today. Mr. Ramirez tells her his wife will be in later. The nurse informs Mr. Ramirez she will work first to get his pain controlled; they can then work together to determine the next interventions. Mr. Ramirez agrees.

The nurse collaborates with the nurse practitioner (NP) on the surgical team regarding Mr. Ramirez's pain control. The NP prescribes a stronger opiate and states he will make rounds later in the morning to assess Mr. Ramirez. He advises the nurse that the pathology report will be available later today; he and the surgeon will meet with Mr. Ramirez and his wife to discuss the results.

The nurse informs Mr. Ramirez of the revised pain management plan and administers the stronger medication. She informs Mr. Ramirez that the NP and surgeon will meet with him and his wife this afternoon. The nurse provides ongoing pain assessment and evaluates the effectiveness of the medication. She coordinates the care provided by other team members to allow Mr. Ramirez to achieve better pain control before increasing his activity. She provides teaching on splinting and breathing techniques to be used to limit pain when getting out of bed and walking. She implements the ordered interventions to prevent complications, including wound care, pulmonary hygiene, and the VTE prevention protocol. The nurse uses increased presence and emotional support to address Mr. Ramirez's anxiety.

Later in the shift, the nurse reviews her documentation of the VTE protocol interventions with the quality improvement nurse specialist and the CNS. Data will be collected to demonstrate effectiveness of the protocol. When the NP and surgeon meet with Mr. Ramirez and his wife, the nurse is present. She remains with Mr. Ramirez and his wife after the news of a positive cancer diagnosis is presented. On the basis of their responses, she revises the plan of care and selects appropriate interventions to meet their needs.

Discussion Topics

1. Discuss how the implementation standards and competencies are demonstrated in this case.

2. Give examples of how nurses coordinate use of resources and the care provided by other disciplines. How does this coordination enhance patient outcomes?

3. How is the importance of sensitivity to diversity demonstrated in the implementation of the standard's competencies?

4. How does the RN demonstrate the competencies in Standard 5B?

5. What guidance do the implementation competencies provide for RNs and APRNs for the use of alternative and complementary therapies?

References and Other Sources

Advanced Practice Registered Nurse Consensus Work Group & the National Council of State Boards of Nursing APRN Advisory Committee (APRN CWG & NCSB). (2008). *Consensus Model for APRN Regulation, Licensure, Accreditation, Certification, and Education*. Retrieved from http://www.aacn.nche.edu/education-resources/APRNReport.pdf

Agency for Healthcare Research and Quality (AHRQ). (2011). *What is comparative-effectiveness research?* Retrieved from http://www.effectivehealthcare.ahrq.gov/index.cfm/what-is-comparative-effectiveness-research1/

Aiken, L. (2008). Effects of hospital care environment on patient mortality outcomes. *The Journal of Nursing Administration, 38*(5), 223–229.

American Association of Critical-Care Nurses (AACN). (2008). *AACN scope and standards for acute and critical care nursing practice*. Aliso Viejo, CA: Author.

American Nurses Association (ANA). (2001). *Code of Ethics for Nurses with interpretative statements*. Washington, DC: American Nurses Publishing.

American Nurses Association (ANA). (2010a). *Nursing's social policy statement: The essence of the profession.* Silver Spring, MD: Nursesbooks .org.

American Nurses Association (ANA). (2010b). *Nursing: Scope and standards of practice* (2nd ed.). Silver Spring, MD: Nursesbooks.org.

Burns, N., & Grove, S. (2007). *Understanding nursing research* (4th ed.). St. Louis, MO: Saunders-Elsevier.

Center for Nursing Classification and Clinical Effectiveness, University of Iowa. (2011). Nursing Outcomes Classification (NOC). Retrieved from http://www.nursing.uiowa.edu/cncce/nursing-outcomes-classification-overview

Institute for Healthcare Improvement (IHI). (2011). *Science of improvement: How to improve.* Retrieved from http://www.ihi.org/knowledge/Pages/HowtoImprove/ScienceofImprovementHowtoImprove.aspx

The Joint Commission. (2011). *Hospital national patient safety goals.* Retrieved from http://www.jointcommission.org/assets/1/6/NPSG_EPs_Scoring_HAP_20110706.pdf

Koloroutis, M. (2004). *Relationship-based care: A model for transforming practice.* Minneapolis, MN: Creative Health Care Management.

Lewin Group. (2011). *What is comparative effectiveness research?* Retrieved from http://www.lewin.com/cer/about/

Potter, P. (2007). Nursing process. In P. Potter & A. Perry (Eds.), *Basic nursing: Essentials for practice.* St. Louis, MO: Mosby.

Potter, P., & Frisch, N. (2009). The holistic caring process. In B. Dossey & L. Keegan (Eds.), *Holistic nursing: A handbook for practice.* Boston, MA: Jones & Bartlett.

Selah, J. (2010). Nursing practice and the nursing process. In S. Nettina (Ed.), *Lippincott manual of nursing practice.* Philadelphia, PA: Wolters Kluwer Health: Lippincott Williams & Wilkins.

Tracy, M. (2009). Direct clinical practice. In A. Hamric, J. Spross, & C. Hanson (Eds.), *Advanced practice nursing: An integrative approach* (4th ed.). St. Louis, MO: Saunders.

The Essential Guide to Nursing Practice

University of Iowa, Center for Nursing Classification and Clinical Effectiveness (n.d.). Nursing Interventions Classification (NIC). Retrieved from http://www.nursing.uiowa.edu/cncce/nursing-interventions-classification-overview

Wilkinson, J. (2007). *Nursing process and critical thinking* (4th ed.). Upper Saddle River, NJ: Pearson Prentice Hall.

Wilkinson, J., & Leuven, K. (2007). *Fundamentals of nursing: Theory, concepts, and applications*. Philadelphia, PA: F. A. Davis.

CHAPTER 9
Standard 6. Evaluation

Janet Y. Harris, MSN, RN, CNAA-BC, and
Kim W. Hoover, PhD, RN

Standard 6. Evaluation. **The registered nurse evaluates progress toward attainment of outcomes.**

Definition and Explanation of the Standard

The evaluation component rounds out the Standards of Practice and the six elements of nursing process: assessment, diagnosis, outcomes identification, planning, implementation, and evaluation. *Evaluation*, the component of interest in this chapter, is defined as "the process of determining the progress toward attainment of expected outcomes, including the effectiveness of care" (ANA, 2010, p. 65). Evaluation is accomplished through direct observation; through interviews with the healthcare consumer, family, and /caregiver; and through reviews of record documentation including progress notes, flow sheets, and results and reports from other departments. In Standard 3, Outcomes Identification, the registered nurse (RN) identifies expected outcomes for a plan individualized to the healthcare consumer or situation. Nurses must create a collective system of accountability by evaluating outcomes through constant evaluation and re-evaluation and adjustment in collaboration with others. Those outcomes may be related to the standards of care, the process of care, or the outcomes of care. Benner, Sutphen, Leonard, and Day (2010) tell us that nurses must ask the right questions, find the right information to answer those questions, and make the best decision on the basis of that information through clinical reasoning. Without the ability to appropriately evaluate, the RN is simply following orders and can potentially cause a breakdown in the entire system of care.

Practice imperatives were established as early as 2001, when the Institute of Medicine (IOM) published *Crossing the Quality Chasm: A New Health System for the 21st Century.* This book called for safe, effective, patient-centered, timely, efficient, and equitable care. The RN and the advanced practice registered nurse (APRN) are critical to the evaluation of those patient outcomes.

The RN provides a systematic, criterion-based evaluation of outcomes prescribed by the plan of care and within the specified time frame. The RN conducts the evaluation in partnership with the healthcare consumer and his or her family or caregivers. The RN also collaborates with other healthcare providers involved with the plan of care to evaluate whether nursing interventions are appropriate and affecting outcomes. During the evaluation, the nurse assesses whether the patient's outcomes have been achieved. The outcomes are met, partially met, or not met at all, and conclusions are drawn about the status of the problem to see if problems are resolved, revised, or continue. The nurse determines if the original diagnoses were correct, if they need to be revised, or if the priorities need to be revisited to meet changing demands. This ongoing assessment determines how well the plan of care is working, if the interventions are effective, if new data are necessary to make the correct evaluation, and if the plan of care needs to be modified. The evaluation depends on all other phases of the nursing process.

The graduate-level prepared specialty nurse and the APRN are expected to evaluate systems more broadly to "determine the effect of the plan on healthcare consumers, families, groups, communities, and institutions" (ANA, 2010, p. 46). Therefore, the advanced practice nurse must evaluate the accuracy of the diagnoses and outcomes demonstrated. Synthesis for those advanced nurses includes a focus on population that includes families, communities, organizations, and systems. Results at this advanced level often focus on policy, process, or protocol revision to affect the larger population of patients or consumers.

Application of the Standard in Practice

Education

Education program standards, outlined by the Commission on Collegiate Nursing Education (CCNE) and the National League for Nursing Accrediting Commission (NLNAC), require that graduate and undergraduate curricula incorporate patient safety and quality improvement content, ranging from using evaluation data to improving patient care while assisting in the design and implementation of new models of care delivery and subsequent evaluation. Criteria listed for nursing practice necessitate an increased level of accountability for APRNs (AACN, 2010a, 2010b, 2011). The National Organization of Nurse Practitioner Faculties (NONPF) competencies include analyzing data, forming an evidence-based action plan, initiating the plan, and evaluating the outcomes of care (NONPF, 2006).

Including a strong component of evaluation in curriculum development, evaluation of students' achievement of learning goals, and evaluation of students by their peers will be aided by evidence-based practice information. This information that can be accessed electronically through reliable sources, such as the Quality and Safety Education for Nurses (QSEN, 2011), which was funded by the Robert Wood Johnson Foundation; the Institute for Healthcare Improvement (IHI, 2011); and the Joanna Briggs Institute (JBI, 2011). A number of tools, such as case studies, standardized patient scenarios, clinical simulation, course content, and electronic health record systems, are available to assist educators teach sound evaluation methods that result in quality improvement. Educators are obligated not only to teach evaluation skills, but also to use them in practice. The use of process improvement tools, including root cause analysis (RCA), models appropriate evaluation standards.

Administration

Structural components of evaluation typically include organizational aspects, such as staffing patterns, risk management structure, reporting mechanisms, and nursing council structure. Each of those components provides opportunities for accountability at broadly defined organizational or unit levels. However, administrative evaluation responsibilities also lie at the individual level where the components are related to processes such as basic competency assessments, job descriptions, performance appraisals, and individual development plans.

Basic competencies, as required by regulatory agencies such as The Joint Commission, must be demonstrated through verification or demonstration of attitude, knowledge, or skill (Wright, 2005). Each organization should define competency and decide how it will be measured. According to Wright, successful competency processes include (1) effectively incorporating competency into daily practice, (2) bundling and communicating the process, (3) managing responses to competency deficits, (4) tracking and documenting the process, and (5) incorporating age-specific cultural criteria and safety into the process. The annual performance review or appraisal is often part of the overall performance assessment along with competency assessment. Work plans become an extension of the appraisal and help set personal and professional development goals for the coming year. The evaluation of those goals is, in turn, included in the evaluative process the following year.

The sources of evidence published in American Nursing Credentialing Center Magnet® documents in 2008 outline the need for Magnet organizations to demonstrate structures and processes that lead to outstanding outcomes. The interaction between core processes and resulting outcomes should be evaluated continually and monitored for improvement. In the description of exemplary professional practice in *Magnet®: The Next Generation—Nurses Making the Difference* (Drenkard, Wolf, & Morgan, 2011), processes should be in place for nurses to use performance- and self-appraisal routinely; this approach should minimally include goal setting and peer review. The center of the Magnet model is titled "empirical outcomes." Nursing-sensitive measures of catheter-associated urinary tract infections and pressure ulcers, measures included in the National Database of Nursing Quality Indicators® (NDNQI®), are examples of outcomes clearly related to nursing care. Through those outcomes, the nurse can evaluate effectiveness of direct patient care (ANA, 2011). In addition, members of the Magnet organization staff should be able to use structures and processes to evaluate existing nursing practices on the basis of evidence.

As a profession, nursing should make significant contributions to patient, nurse, and organizational outcomes regardless of the environment in which care is delivered. Myriad providers, managers, administrators, and organizational leaders should continually monitor the relationships between structures, processes, and outcomes. Some frequently evaluated outcomes for patients include hospital- or system-acquired infections, such as central line blood stream infections or catheter-associated urinary tract infections, falls and injuries associated with falls, hospital-acquired pressure ulcers, and the patient's perception of safety. Nurse satisfaction and engagement, turnover, and staff perception of the work environment are a few examples of nurse-specific outcomes. Efficiency and effectiveness constitute organizational outcomes, while the effect of community outreach programs and community wellness serve as examples for patient outcomes.

Performance and Quality Improvement

A number of healthcare improvement gurus, including Paul Batalden and Donald Berwick, have been credited with the phrase "every system is perfectly designed to get exactly the results it gets" (Carr, 2008). No matter the origin, this statement compels us to include hardwire evaluation as part of our individual and collective healthcare practice systems so that we may improve practice and meet the six aims for an improved healthcare system: safe, timely, effective, efficient, equitable, and patient-centered (IOM, 2001). The emphasis on quality improvement in health care today demands that evaluation data are used to improve patient care and to prevent complications, referred to as hospital-acquired conditions or potentially preventable complications. In a review of Magnet outcome literature, Lundmark and Hickey (Drenkard, Wolf, & Morgan, 2011) found that individual nurses working collectively can improve systems of care. Evidence-based practice and research standards are clearly linked to evaluation. Organizations must rely on nonpunitive risk mitigation, thereby concentrating on "good catches" rather than "near misses."

Research

When evaluation of measurable outcomes becomes hardwired into nursing practice, we create a culture of inquiry that results in better evidence for practice. An example of an established nursing-sensitive indicator database is the NDNQI database, which was spearheaded by ANA to create a national database from which nurses could learn collectively. Nursing-led research continues to grow, particularly in hospitals with Magnet status, but building nursing research capacity depends on the systematic collection of individual evaluation data regarding practice, no matter the setting. Collection of appropriate data is supported through the nurse's perusal of current knowledge, translation of that knowledge into practice, evaluation of the effectiveness of those practices, and subsequent inquiry into better patient care.

Conclusion

Standard 6 Evaluation describes the expectation that the RN evaluates progress toward attainment of outcomes. This final step in the nursing process requires competence in conducting a systematic, ongoing, and criterion-based evaluation of the outcomes in relation to the structures and processes prescribed by the plan and indicated timeline. Collaboration with the healthcare consumer and others involved in the care or situation is an essential component of the evaluation process. Ongoing assessment data inform revision of the diagnoses, outcomes, plan, and implementation as needed.

Case Studies and Discussion Topics

Case Study 1

You are the only RN in a hospital pediatric unit with 10 patients. Two nursing assistants and one nurse extern are on the unit. You have two patients who are 10 to 12 hours post-operative. One 13-year-old patient had minor surgery but is mentally disabled and has trouble communicating. The other patient, an 8-year-old, had abdominal surgery and is alert and responsive.

1. Using the pain assessment, intervention, and reassessment or response (AIR) cycle, how might you evaluate both patients differently to determine if pain management is achieved?

2. Develop a plan for evaluating pain management to use during your 12-hour shift that includes other members of your shift team.

Case Study 2

You are the nurse practitioner director of an urban clinic in an underserved metropolitan area. In an attempt to influence the health of your teenage clients, you have been speaking to all of them about risky health behaviors, but you recognize that many are not adhering to recommendations because they see those behaviors as the norm. You decide that the best way to influence the community is to seek grant funding for a community action plan. However, you know the funders will consider only plans with strong evaluation components that include empirical outcomes. You want to begin by addressing teenage pregnancy in partnership with local organizations.

1. What interventions would you consider?

2. What short- and long-term measurable outcomes would you include in your proposal?

References and Other Sources

American Nurses Association (ANA). (2010). *Nursing: Scope and standards of practice* (2nd ed.). Silver Spring, MD: Nursesbooks.org.

American Nurses Association (ANA). (2011). National Database of Nursing Quality Indicators®. Retrieved from https://www.nursingquality.org/

American Association of Colleges of Nursing (AACN). (2008). *The essentials of baccalaureate education for professional nursing practice.* Washington, DC: Author. Retrieved from http://www.aacn.nche.edu/education/pdf/BaccEssentials08.pdf

American Association of Colleges of Nursing (AACN). (2010a). *Leveling grids for AACN baccalaureate, master's, and DNP essentials.* Washington, DC: Author. Retrieved from http://www.aan.nche.edu/Faculty/FacultyLink/pdf/MastersEssentialsGrids.pdf

American Association of Colleges of Nursing (AACN). (2010b). *The essentials for doctoral education in advanced practice nursing.* Washington, DC: Author. Retrieved from http://www.aacn.nche.edu/DNP/pdf/Essentials.pdf

American Association of Colleges of Nursing (AACN). (2011). *The essentials of master's education in nursing.* Washington, DC: Author. Retrieved from http://www.aacn.nche.edu/education/pdf/Master'sEssentials11.pdf

Benner, P., Sutphen, M., Leonard, V., & Day, L. (2010). Educating nurses: A call for radical transformation. San Francisco, CA: Jossey-Bass.

Carr, S. (2008, July/August). Editor's notebook: A quotation with a life of its own. *Patient Safety & Quality Healthcare.* Retrieved from http://www.psqh.com/julaug08/editor.html

Drenkard, K., Wolf, G., & Morgan, S. (Eds.). (2011). *Magnet®: The next generation—Nurses making the difference.* Silver Spring, MD: American Nurses Credentialing Center.

Institute for Healthcare Improvement. (2011). Retrieved from http://www.ihi.org/ihi

Institute of Medicine (IOM). (2001). *Crossing the quality chasm: A new health system for the 21st century.* Washington, DC: National Academies Press.

Joanna Briggs Institute. (2011). Retrieved from http://www.joannabriggs.edu.au/

Lundmark, V., & Hickey, J. (2011). Magnet practice environments and outcomes. In K. Drenkard, G. Wolf, & S. Morgan (Eds.), *Magnet®: The next generation—Nurses making the difference* (pp. 115–139). Silver Spring, MD: American Nurses Credentialing Center.

Luquire, R., & Strong, M. (2011). Empirical outcomes. In K. Drenkard, G. Wolf, & S. Morgan (Eds.), *Magnet®: The next generation—Nurses making the difference* (pp. 93–103). Silver Spring, MD: American Nurses Credentialing Center.

National Organization of Nurse Practitioner Faculties (NONPF). (2006). Domains and core competencies of nurse practitioner practice. Washington, DC: NONPF. Retrieved from http://www.nonpf.com/associations/10789/files/DomainsandCoreComps2006.pdf

Quality and Safety Education for Nurses (QSEN). (2011). Princeton, NJ: Robert Wood Johnson Foundation. Retrieved from http://www.qsen.org

Wright, D. (2005). *The ultimate guide to competency assessment in health care* (2nd ed., rev.). Minneapolis, MN: Creative Health Care Management, Inc.

CHAPTER 10

Standard 7. Ethics

Linda L. Olson, PhD, RN, NEA-BC

Standard 7. Ethics. **The registered nurse practices ethically.**

Definition and Explanation of the Standard

Although ethics is considered a distinct and separate standard of professional performance, it is a concept that is an inherent component of all of the standards of professional practice and performance, as well as across all nursing roles and settings. *Code of Ethics for Nurses with Interpretive Statements* (ANA, 2001) is the ethical standard and framework for the nursing profession. The document guides nurses who encounter everyday ethical issues as well as more challenging ethical situations such as end-of-life decisions. Ethics occur within the context of relationships with others. The relationships include those of nurse to healthcare consumer, nurse to physician, nurse to other members of the interprofessional team, nurse to nurse, nurse to employer, nurse to profession, nurse to nursing students, and nurse to society. The concept of ethics also occurs within the context of nurses' personal and professional values and the core values of the profession.

The Code of Ethics for Nurses, which has evolved over time, is a dynamic document that is revised periodically to remain current with the advances in the profession and in the healthcare environment. The Code reflects the profession's central and enduring values, which include service to and duties toward those for whom we care, as well as to ourselves. The values of the profession provide a frame of reference for priority setting and for ethical decision-making.

Those shared professional values are inherent in the profession's code of ethics. In contrasting the profession's ethical standard with its legal standard (nurse practice acts), actions that are ethical may not be considered to be legal. In turn, what is legal may not be perceived as being ethical and may be in conflict with one's personal values. The Code of Ethics for Nurses is a resource for nurses when faced with difficult situations.

As stated in the Code of Ethics for Nurses, "ethics is an integral part of the foundation of nursing" (ANA, 2001, p. 5). This foundation, by which the nursing profession fulfills its commitment to serve the interests of society by embracing and acting according to a strong code of ethics, is an integral component of nursing's social contract (ANA, 2010a, p. 5). In whatever role or setting, nurses share a commitment to ethical practice and to service as ethical role models for others. Nursing's relationship with patients (whether an individual, family, group, or community receiving nursing care and services) is based on the social contract between society and the profession.

The terms *ethics* and *morals* are often used interchangeably. *Morality* usually refers to one's personal behavior related to distinguishing right from wrong. Although *ethics* are central to the concept of morality when making ethical choices and decisions, one often must choose between options where there is more than one right choice or where there are equally less than acceptable choices. Many of the ethical issues encountered daily by nurses relate to protecting the rights of patients and families, upholding their autonomy, ensuring informed consent, and assisting patients and families in the expression of self-determination such as advanced directive decisions. Nurses also confront legal and regulatory issues, such as deciding when and how to question inappropriate behaviors of other healthcare professionals or practices that affect the quality of patient care and safety. Those issues, along with others associated with safe staffing and its effect on quality of care, are associated with caregiver stress, job satisfaction, and retention (Ulrich et al., 2010). Having the ability to deal effectively with such everyday ethical issues—in addition to the more serious life-and-death and end-of-life issues—comprises the competencies that nurses must possess as part of the professional performance standard that is related to ethics. In turn, administrators in practice settings where nurses work are responsible for creating healthy work environments by providing adequate resources and organizational mechanisms such as ethics committees, consultants, and education to assist nurses who address ethical concerns.

In the standard of professional performance related to ethics, several competencies identify the nurse's role in advocating for—and protecting the rights of—those for whom we care and provide services, whether they are individuals, family members, communities, groups, systems, or other stakeholders. Additional competencies include participation in interdisciplinary teams and in organizational mechanisms that address and inform ethical decisions and outcomes. Collaboration with others in influencing resource allocation and in advocating for patients is itself an ethical process.

Application of the Standard in Practice

Ethical nursing practice, as a part of the foundation of nursing, provides the basis for nurses' commitment to society to provide and ensure safe and quality patient care. In doing so, nurses in all areas of practice settings and roles demonstrate the value that society places in the profession. Over the past several years, the annual Gallup poll survey about honesty and ethics in professions has placed nurses at the top.

Education

In pre-licensure nursing education, students need to learn how to recognize the existence of an ethical issue (ethical awareness), as well as how to think about and reason about ethical situations (ethical reflection, reasoning, and decision-making), and then how to determine the most appropriate action. Students need to identify and have insight into their personal and professional values (which are learned and cultivated throughout their life experiences with family, friends, and religion) and then to be able to identify how their personal values relate to the values of the profession and their relationship to patients. Ways of accomplishing these goals include having courses on ethics and ethical reasoning, as well as integrating ethics and ethical principles throughout all levels of nursing curriculum and in the clinical arena. In the current multicultural society, students also need to learn about the values and ethics of the various cultural groups with whom they interact, the issue of ethical boundaries, and the appropriate use of mechanisms of communication (i.e., social media). As nurses advance in their careers, they are responsible for lifelong learning and maintenance of their professional and clinical competence. Maintaining continued competence is an ethical responsibility of professional nurses and an expectation of the society to which nurses are accountable.

As emphasized in the report from the Carnegie Foundation for the Advancement of Teaching's study on nursing education (Benner, Sutphen, Leonard, & Day, 2010), nurses must develop ethical competence and a sense of ethical comportment. Everyday ethical comportment includes the appropriate use of knowledge and skills to provide care to patients, using effective communication and interpersonal skills with patients and colleagues, as well as the ability to engage in ethical reflection. Also, behaving ethically encompasses the ability to respond to errors in a transparent, ethical way so that learning can occur and future episodes can be avoided. By serving as role models for ethical comportment, faculty members can help students to think ethically about their care of patients, thus using moral imagination, which then results in enhancing their ethical responsibility (Benner et al., 2010). As role models, faculty members are expected to treat their colleagues with respect and to be open and willing to listen, to value, and to respect diverse viewpoints, as well as to effectively deal with conflict.

Administration

Recently, business and healthcare literature has emphasized the importance of ethical leadership. An ethical leader possesses the qualities of self-knowledge, personal integrity, and the ability to serve as a role model. A component of ethical leadership is the ability to coach and mentor others. Transformational leaders foster personal and professional development in others. They stimulate innovation, creativity, and appropriate risk-taking through the process of mutual engagement. Another component of ethical leadership is fairness, which includes being open and honest in understanding and considering the viewpoints of others and in assisting others to express their views on issues without fear of reprisal or other consequences. One of the most important aspects of ethical leadership is trust plus the creation of relationships in which the leader is viewed as trustworthy, as well as having the ability to trust that others will feel free to express their opinions and to act in ways that promote the best interests of the patients. Ethical leaders are responsible for creating a healthy, positive workplace environment. If one is to do this, mechanisms should be in place for nurses and others to access ethics advice and consultation, written policies related to dealing with ethical issues and concerns, and education and formats for discussion of ethical issues and concerns. A component of ethics education is ensuring that nurses are aware of and knowledgeable about the content of the Code of Ethics for Nurses. Such mechanisms encourage an open awareness and discussion of ethical issues.

Many institutions are implementing the concept of Just Culture, which improves patient safety by creating a work culture that promotes an open and fair mechanism for reporting patient errors and near misses (ANA, 2010c; Marx, 2001). This concept has become incorporated into performance evaluation, quality improvement, patient safety, and risk management programs in many hospitals.

With the growth of electronic media as mechanisms for increasing access by students to nursing education through the use of online learning, the use of electronic medical records, and the use of social media in both personal and professional communication, there is an increase in the frequency and type of ethical issues that surface. The electronic means of communication create increased demands on the role of the registered nurse (and the nursing student) in protecting patient privacy and confidentiality. Simply refraining from discussing patients and their situations in public spaces is no longer adequate. Discussing or revealing patient information through mobile phones and cameras, the Internet, and social networking sites constitutes a breach of patient confidentiality and privacy. Those technologies have created new and emerging sources of ethical dilemmas. In addition, there are legal implications related to potential violations of the Health Insurance Portability and Accountability Act (HIPAA).

Performance and Quality Improvement

Nurses in all roles and settings are expected to engage in activities that create a culture of continuous quality improvement and patient safety. The Hastings Center, in its reports on quality improvement, takes the position that all healthcare providers, including individuals as well as institutions, are ethically responsible for managing and continuously improving the quality of services they deliver (Baily, Bottrell, Lynn, & Jennings, 2006; Jennings, Baily, Bottrell, & Lynn, 2007). The aim of quality improvement (QI) activities is to identify opportunities to improve the delivery of healthcare services, to learn from mistakes, and to produce benefits and improved outcomes for patients in a timely manner. Therefore, those activities must be conducted in an ethically responsible and systematic way that protects patients from harm and promotes benefits for patients and providers.

By basing their clinical decision-making and nursing interventions on the best available evidence and by using QI methods to assess patient outcomes, nurses contribute to quality as well as cost-effective patient care. Graduate-level specialty prepared nurses and advanced practice registered nurses (APRNs), such as nurse practitioners, clinical nurse specialists, certified nurse midwives, and certified registered nurse anesthetists, have unique roles in using their knowledge and skills to contribute to quality patient outcomes and to evaluate the effectiveness of nursing interventions. In addition, the supportive role of nurse executives and nurse managers, along with their role in creating a culture that facilitates continuous quality improvement and research, is key to promoting and contributing to safe, effective, and quality patient outcomes.

There has been debate on the issue of whether QI projects should meet the rigorous approval requirements of an institutional review board (IRB) to which research projects adhere. Results of QI projects are expected to be incorporated into changes in institutional policies and practices more rapidly than are the results of the more rigorous scientific research studies. Generally, IRB approval is not required for QI projects unless the results will be published or the projects have the potential for exposing patients to harm (Shirey et al., 2010).

Research

The aim of nursing research is to generate new knowledge and add to the body of knowledge of nursing science. Nurses who conduct and participate in research are responsible for ensuring that the rights of human subjects are protected through appropriate review by IRBs. This ethical review of proposed research protects the public by giving assurance that research participants both receive information about the risks and benefits of the research and provide their informed consent; that their participation is voluntary; and that anonymity and confidentiality are maintained. Doctorally prepared nurses and APRNs are especially encouraged to add to the body of nursing science by generating new knowledge through research, as well as by mentoring others in learning about and participating in the research process.

Evidence-based practice (EBP) is another mechanism for promoting quality patient care. EBP focuses on finding and using the best available evidence as the basis for decision-making and patient care interventions. It bases nursing practice and changes in nursing practice on the strength of the available evidence, while also keeping patient preferences and values in mind. Using the best available evidence as the basis for patient care interventions results in better patient care outcomes and is a component of the ethical practice of nursing. If strong evidence is not available to implement a practice change, the nurse has an ethical responsibility to carry out additional research.

Conclusion

As members of the nursing profession who are accountable to the public for their practice, nurses are expected to comply with the scope and professional standards of nursing practice, including the ethics standard. However, ethics is a concept that is inherent in all standards of professional practice and performance. Ethical practice is a component of the role of nurses across all settings and educational backgrounds. The Code of Ethics for Nurses is the profession's nonnegotiable standard and framework. Along with the Scope of Practice and the Professional Standards of Nursing Practice, the Code of Ethics for Nurses provides guidance to nurses when faced with difficult ethical issues, problems, or dilemmas.

Case Study and Discussion Topics

Case Study

The following is a hypothetical situation that demonstrates the role of the nurse in serving as a patient advocate:

- The staff nurse turns to ethics consultation to meet the best interests of the identified patient. The nurse accesses resources in the hospital to help make decisions when conflicts about treatment options for patients occur among care providers and family members. The staff nurse turns to ethics consultation to meet the best interests of the identified patient. Nurses owe the same duties to themselves as to others. Recognizing this responsibility, the nurse manager serves as an advocate for the staff nurse. This approach also upholds commitment to the best interests of the patient, because research has shown an increased potential for errors and a negative impact on patient safety when nurses are fatigued.

- A critical-care nurse in a medical intensive care unit in an inner city has spent a busy 12-hour night shift working with a critically ill patient (and family) who is receiving advanced treatments. The patient's prognosis is poor. At the end of the shift, the nurse informs the nurse manager of the issues that have occurred during the night and requests an ethics consult. The nurse manager listens carefully to the staff nurse, who is visibly distraught over the situation in which she feels the patient's expressed desires are not being respected. Also, the nurse tells the manager that a nurse on the next shift has called in sick and that she is willing to stay during the day to cover the unit. The manager informs the staff nurse that she will follow up on the request for an ethics consult, but that she cannot approve the staff nurse's request for overtime (even though she would like to). The manager knows that research-based evidence has shown that nurses who are fatigued and who work more than 12 hours at a time are at greater risk for patient errors (Lorenz, 2008; Rogers, Hwang, Scott, Aiken, & Dinges, 2004; Trinkoff et al., 2011).

This case demonstrates a staff nurse serving as a patient advocate. It also represents the nurse manager's role as advocate for staff members by acknowledging that nurses have not only a duty to patients, but also a duty to self. According to hospital policy, any nurse who has an ethics concern about patient care is authorized to call an ethics consult. This mechanism is part of the organization's culture and reflects a commitment to assist nurses with challenging ethical issues. As a part of the organization's climate, the ethical climate is a positive one as perceived by nurses (Olson, 1998). Nurses feel empowered to ask for a consultation when faced with difficult ethical issues. They perceive that mechanisms are within the workplace to help them to reflect on, discuss, and make decisions that contribute to their ethical practice. In addition, their professional relationships with the interprofessional team, the patient, and other stakeholders demonstrate respect for and openness to diverse viewpoints.

Discussion Topics

1. Identify an ethical issue you have faced either with a patient or a colleague. How would you use the information about the professional standard on ethics and the Code of Ethics for Nurses to help you understand the issue? What are some ways to resolve the issue?

2. Discuss the concepts of ethical practice and ethical leadership.

3. What kinds of mechanisms in the workplace environment serve to help nurses when faced with difficult and challenging patient care issues?

4. Identify an ethical issue related to your scope of practice as an RN, student nurse, or APRN. Find a position statement of a professional nursing organization related to this issue (e.g., the role of the nurse in end-of-life decisions).

5. Ethics is an essential component of the scope and standards of practice and of professionalism. Discuss this concept in relation to your own practice.

References and Other Sources

American Nurses Association (ANA). (2001). *Code of Ethics for Nurses with interpretive statements.* Washington, DC: American Nurses Publishing.

American Nurses Association (ANA). (2010a). *Nursing's social policy statement: The essence of the profession.* Silver Spring, MD: Nursesbooks .org.

American Nurses Association (ANA). (2010b). *Nursing: Scope and standards of practice* (2nd ed.). Silver Spring, MD: Nursesbooks.org.

American Nurses Association (ANA). (2010c). Just culture. ANA position statement. Silver Spring, MD: Author.

Baily, M. A., Bottrell, M., Lynn, J., & Jennings, B. (2006). *The ethics of using QI methods to improve health care quality and safety.* New York, NY: The Hastings Center.

Benefiel, D. (2011). The story of nurse licensure. *Nurse Educator, 36*(1), 16–20.

Benner, P., Sulphen, M., Leonard, V., & Day, L. (2010). *Educating nurses: A call for radical transformation.* San Francisco, CA: Jossey-Bass.

Fowler, M. (Ed.). (2008). *Guide to the Code of Ethics for Nurses: Interpretation and application.* Silver Spring, MD: Nursesbooks.org.

Institute of Medicine. (IOM) (2011). *The future of nursing: Leading change, advancing health.* Washington, DC: National Academies Press.

Jennings, B., Baily, M. A., Bottrell, M., & Lynn, J. (2007). *Health care quality improvement: Ethical and regulatory issues.* New York, NY: The Hastings Center.

Lorenz, S. G. (2008). 12-hour shifts: An ethical dilemma for the nurse executive. *Journal of Nursing Administration, 38*(6), 297–301.

Marx, D. (2001). *Patient safety and the "just culture": A primer for health care executives.* New York, NY: Columbia University.

Olson, L. L. (1998). Hospital nurses' perceptions of the ethical climate of their work setting. *Journal of Nursing Scholarship, 30*(4), 345–349.

Pavlish, C., Brown-Saltzman, K., Hersh, M., Shirk, M., & Nudelman, O. (2011). Early indicators and risk factors for ethical issues in clinical practice. *Journal of Nursing Scholarship, 43*(1), 13–21.

Rogers, A. E., Hwang, W. T., Scott, L. D., Aiken, L. H., & Dinges, D. F. (2004). The working hours of hospital staff nurses and patient safety. *Health Affairs, 23*(4), 202–212.

Shirey, M. R., Hauck, S. L., Embree, J. L., Kinner, T. J., Schaar, G. L., Phillips, L. A., Ashby, S. R., Swenty, C. F., & McCool, I. A. (2010). Showcasing differences between quality improvement, evidence-based practice, and research. *The Journal of Continuing Education in Nursing, 20*(10), 1–12.

Trinkoff, A. M., Johantgen, M., Storr, C. L., Gurses, A. P., Liang, Y., & Han, K. (2011). Nurses' work schedule characteristics, nurse staffing, and patient mortality. *Nursing Research, 60*(1), 1–8.

Ulrich, C. M., Taylor, C., Soeken, K., O'Donnell, P., Farrar, A., Danis, M., & Grady, C. (2010). Everyday ethics: Ethical issues and stress in nursing practice. *Journal of Advanced Nursing, 66*(11), 2510–2519.

CHAPTER 11

Standard 8. Education

Pamela A. Kulbok, DNSc, RN, PHCNS-BC, FAAN

Standard 8. Education. **The registered nurse attains knowledge and competence that reflects current nursing practice.**

Definition and Explanation of the Standard

The professional practice of nursing is dynamic. It constantly evolves and responds to the emerging health and illness needs of individuals, families, communities, and populations; to the rapid advances in science and technology; and to the continual changes in healthcare systems and policies (ANA, 2010a). There has been long-standing recognition that current, effective, and safe nursing practice requires a unique body of knowledge (Risjord, 2010). Nursing knowledge for clinical practice is derived from nursing science and the biopsychosocial, economic, organizational, political, and technological sciences. Nurses apply theory-based and evidence-based knowledge in a collaborative process with patients and others to provide high-quality care and to produce positive, quality health outcomes (ANA, 2010b). The education Standard of Professional Performance describes the professional obligation to acquire and maintain the knowledge and competencies necessary for current nursing practice (ANA, 2010a).

Education is requisite for acquisition of the knowledge, skills, and abilities needed to maintain current, safe, and effective clinical practice. The ability to acquire, appraise, and apply the best scientific evidence in nursing practice is sustained through ongoing professional education. Melnyk and Fineout-Overholt (2005, p. 5) remind us that "without current best evidence, practice is rapidly outdated, often to the detriment of patients."

The recent release of report titled *The Future of Nursing: Leading Change, Advancing Health* by the Institute of Medicine (IOM, 2011) posited four key messages to develop an action-oriented blueprint with recommendations for the future of nursing. One of those messages was specific to nursing education: Nurses should achieve higher levels of education and training through an improved education system that promotes seamless academic progression.

Both formal and informal learning opportunities for nursing have expanded dramatically in recent years. Formal educational opportunities at the graduate level include new programs such as master's entry clinical nurse leader (CNL) programs, numerous graduate nursing specialties, and the doctor of nursing practice (DNP) degree. There are multiple paths to registered nurse (RN) licensure and a professional nursing career, including a diploma, an associate degree, and a baccalaureate degree. Despite the nurse's entry into nursing practice pathway, obtaining knowledge and competencies to meet emerging health and illness needs of individuals, families, communities, and populations and the ever-changing healthcare system requires educational advancement beyond the associate degree or diploma level (Creasia & Reid, 2011). Professional education is also available in diverse nursing practice environments through structured educational activities such as orientation and in-service, continuing education, and other career development programs. Nursing certification in a role, population, or specialty is also available to validate the acquisition of additional skills, knowledge, and abilities through advanced education or specialized training.

Professional nursing practice at both the generalist and graduate levels must keep pace with progress in health care and, by virtue of the profession's social contract with the public, must meet standards of competence for professional behavior delineated by professional and specialty nursing organizations (ANA, 2010a, 2010b). There are 10 competencies—or measurable expectations—for the education Standard of Professional Performance for RNs and one competency for graduate-level prepared specialty nurses or advanced practice registered nurses (APRNs) (ANA, 2010a). Education competencies for RNs include both formal and informal approaches, such as continuing education focused on the growing evidence base for clinical nursing practice, as well as a personal commitment to lifelong learning, self-assessment, and inquiry to maintain professional growth.

Continuing education and lifelong learning involve actively seeking educational opportunities to improve clinical practice performance and acquiring knowledge and skills appropriate to nurses' specific professional roles, target populations, specialties, practice settings, or situations. Formal learning experiences also include academic advancement, that is, from Associate Degree in Nursing (ADN) to a Bachelor of Science in Nursing (BSN) degree or to a Master of Science in Nursing (MSN) or from a BSN to a master's or doctoral degree. Such formal learning is also intended to help a nurse acquire and maintain specialized skills and knowledge. Registered nurses demonstrate competence in education by identifying their learning needs on the basis of new nursing knowledge, professional roles they may assume, career goals, and shifting population needs. They may participate in consultations to address practice issues and share new knowledge, experiences, and ideas with co-workers. RNs contribute to a work environment that is conducive to education for healthcare professionals, and they maintain professional records that provide evidence of competence and lifelong learning.

Graduate-level prepared specialty nurses or APRNs are expected to demonstrate the competencies appropriate for all RNs. In addition, they apply current research and other evidence to expand their clinical knowledge, skills, abilities, and judgment; to enhance their role performance; and to increase knowledge of professional issues.

Application of the Standard in Practice

Education
Personal and professional self-assessment is necessary to identify formal and informal learning opportunities, within and beyond the practice environment, that provide the knowledge and competencies necessary for the provision of current, high-quality nursing and health care. Self-assessment is a component of reflective learning, which involves thoughtful personal analysis and synthesis of areas of strength and capacity for improvement (ANA, 2008). Through self-assessment activities, nurses across roles and specialties identify gaps in their knowledge and skills that can be addressed by targeted professional development and continuing education (CE) programs. In addition, the process of self-assessment and reflective analysis may lead nurses to seek specialty certification, which acknowledges acquisition of advanced knowledge, skills, and abilities.

Continuing education is a traditional form of education designed to promote personal and professional growth and to stay up-to-date with new developments in health care. In a recent article on dissemination of cancer education,

Ousley, Swarz, Milliken, and Ellis (2010) emphasize the challenges of translating new evidence into clinical practice; that is, it may take up to 17 years for scientific innovation and new knowledge to reach the bedside. In addition, Ousley et al. (2010) point out that the most effective forms of CE that are likely to achieve behavior change for healthcare providers will use multiple, interactive learning methods. Currently, 18 states require CE to maintain RN licensure (Gannett Healthcare Group, 2011). There are several deterrents to nurses' participation in CE programs and professional development, including "the cost of attending CE, inability to get time off from work, and child care and home responsibilities" (Schweitzer & Krassa, 2010, p. 443). Increased awareness of those barriers by CE providers and employers may enhance future CE opportunities. Moreover, professional nurses must understand the importance of continuing education and must seek opportunities for growth and development within a focus area, role, or specialty of nursing.

The American Board of Nursing Specialties (ABNS) defined certification as a form of recognition for nurses who gain specialized knowledge, skills, and abilities and who demonstrate the achievement of standards established by nursing specialty organizations (Styles, Schumann, Bickford, & White, 2008). Certification validates the acquisition of advanced knowledge through education and clinical experience. In 2005, the ABNS collected data on the perceived value of nursing specialty certification from certified nurses, noncertified nurses, and nursing managers. Overall, the study participants validated statements on the intrinsic and extrinsic value of nursing specialty certification (Niebuhr & Biel, 2007). According to the American Nurses Credentialing Center (ANCC, 2011a), "board certification and recognition empowers nurses within their professional sphere of activity and contributes to better patient outcomes." CE is one form of professional development that partially fulfills the requirements for graduate-level specialty recertification conferred by ANCC (2011b). As of January 1, 2014, the ANCC recertification process for all applicants will require 75 CE hours every 5 years. In light of those facts, RNs and graduate-level nurses need to be proactive and to assume personal responsibility for continuing education and lifelong learning so they maintain current clinical practice.

Administration

A basic education competency for all professional nurses is to contribute to a practice environment that is conducive to the education of healthcare professionals. Nursing administrators have specific responsibilities for fostering a healthy work environment that provides opportunities for staff development through formal and informal learning and education. Within the context of a healthy work environment, performance appraisal is another application of the education Standard of Professional Performance and competencies. For example, competency-based performance appraisal tools have been developed and tested for use in public health nursing (PHN) (Kalb et al., 2006). The PHN competencies (Quad Council of Public Health Nursing Organizations, 2004) provided a useful framework for developing a performance appraisal tool for five nursing practice classifications—staff RN, public health nurse, nurse practitioner, clinical nurse specialist, and nursing supervisor—in an urban public health department. The performance appraisal tool was used to provide meaningful feedback to nursing employees and to facilitate genuine communication between employees and supervisors.

Performance appraisal can also be viewed as an important element of quality assurance and improvement processes (Smith, Gunzenhauser, & Fielding, 2010). An employer can use performance appraisal or evaluation to assess an employee's knowledge, competencies, and adherence to professional standards. Smith et al. (2010) used best practices for performance evaluation to overcome challenges and negative attitudes related to evaluating employee's performance in a local health department. The keys to building a fair and effective evaluation process involved the employees in annual goal-setting, in using agreed-upon competencies, in clear and role-specific statements of duties or tasks, and in consistent standards of practice. The public health nurses took responsibility and participated in evaluating their performance, knowledge, and competencies according to clear behavioral expectations.

Performance and Quality Improvement

Another valuable method of self-assessment and evaluation of nursing knowledge and practice competencies is the use of a professional portfolio. A portfolio is a form of documentation of intentional or proactive professional development, with the specific goal of attaining knowledge and competence that reflects current, effective, and safe nursing practice. A portfolio is more than a resume or curriculum vitae. It is a collection of the evidence and materials further informed by one's reflection on the meanings of the underlying experiences, which document a nurse's competencies over time. Moreover, those materials may reflect the "background, skills, and expertise of the nurse" (Oermann, 2002, p. 73). According to Oermann (2002), there are two forms of portfolios: one form documents exemplary achievements and expertise (i.e., best work for review by others), and the other is a working document for personal use to record and evaluate professional learning, (i.e., growth and development). Portfolios may include a wide range of evidence and material, such as a resume, 5-year goals, formal academic transcripts, CE certificates, position descriptions, clinical presentations, executive summaries of completed projects, and publications.

Research

Research in 2003 by Aiken, Clarke, Cheung, Sloane, and Silber on the levels of education of hospital nurses and mortality of surgical patients has been called "groundbreaking" and illustrated "one very simple point: education makes a difference in nursing practice" (Long, 2004, p. 48). In a study of more than 230,000 surgical discharges from 168 nonfederal adult general hospitals in Pennsylvania, Aiken and colleagues found that "a 10% increase in the proportion of nurses holding a bachelor's degree [in hospitals] was associated with a 5% decrease in both the likelihood of patients dying within 30 days of admission and the odds of failure to rescue [deaths in patients with serious complications]" (Aiken et al., 2003, p. 1617). More recently, while using the data from the same sources as the Aiken study, Kutney-Lee and Aiken (2008) reported that length of stay was shorter for surgical patients with serious mental illness in hospitals where nurses had more education.

Brooten, Youngblut, Kutcher, and Bobo (2004) reviewed research demonstrating an association between advanced practice nursing (APN) and quality health care. The authors examined a series of studies supporting a positive effect of APN "dose" (i.e., time per patient, patient outcomes, and cost of health care). For example, improved pregnancy outcomes and decreased costs were reported in a randomized trial of in-home prenatal care provided by nurse specialists with master's degrees (Brooten et al., 2001). Although more research is warranted, evidence is accruing that having a baccalaureate and higher education makes a difference in high-quality health care.

Conclusion

The education Standard of Professional Performance delineates the professional obligation of registered nurses and graduate-level prepared specialty nurses or APRNs to acquire and maintain the knowledge and competencies essential for current, effective, and safe nursing practice (ANA, 2010a). Formal and informal education and lifelong learning are requisite for professional nursing practice that is responsive to the complex emerging healthcare needs of individuals, families, communities, and populations. Formal and informal education and lifelong learning provide the foundation for current, up-to-date, theory-based, and evidence-based professional practice in continually evolving nursing roles, specialties, and practice environments. The ability of registered nurses and graduate-level prepared specialty nurses or APRNs to provide quality care and to produce positive, quality health outcomes depends on acquisition, appraisal, and application of the best scientific evidence through ongoing personal and professional education.

Case Study and Discussion Topics

Case Study

Marie is a recent graduate of a DNP program where she focused on women's health care and prevention of intimate partner violence. Her personal story of professional growth and development throughout her nursing career reflects the essence of the education professional performance standard. Marie began her professional nursing career with an ADN. She worked on an internal medicine unit of a university health system for several years, and, during that time, she completed her BSN degree by studying part-time. While completing her BSN program, she was required to create a professional portfolio to track her career development and to set goals for future advancement. When she graduated from her BSN program, she became a member of the American Nurses Association.

As Marie was advancing on the career ladder within the health system, she became more interested in women's health issues and requested a transfer to an obstetrics and gynecology unit. To increase her knowledge and skills in obstetrics nursing, she completed several in-service and career development programs offered within her health system, as well as CE courses. Within a few years, she enrolled in an MSN degree program. During her MSN program, she became interested in domestic violence, particularly intimate partner violence during pregnancy. She sought information on specialized training in this area and became certified as a Sexual Assault Nurse Examiner (SANE). Marie aspired to grow and advance in the nursing profession. At the same time, she wanted to remain clinically proficient and to continue to practice at the bedside. She learned about the DNP degree while studying for her master's degree. She saw the DNP as an opportunity to advance to the highest level of clinical practice.

Discussion Topics

The future looks bright for Marie, her patients, nursing colleagues, and health-care collaborators.

- How has Marie's story influenced you?

- What opportunities do you see for advancement in your specialty area?

- What strategies can you use to document your professional growth and development?

- What role does education serve as you plan your 5-year career goals?

References and Other Sources

Aiken, L. H., Cheung, R. B., & Olds, D. M. (2009). Education policy initiatives to address the nurse shortage in the United States. *Health Affairs, 28*(4), 646–656.

Aiken, L. H., Clarke, S. P., Cheung, R. B., Sloane D. M., & Silber, J. H. (2003). Educational levels of hospital nurses and surgical patient mortality. *JAMA, 290*(12), 1617–1623.

American Nurses Association (ANA). (2008). *Professional role competence* (Position Statement). Silver Spring, MDs: Author.

American Nurses Association (ANA). (2010a). *Nursing: Scope and standards of practice* (2nd ed.). Silver Spring, MD: Nursesbooks.org.

American Nurses Association (ANA). (2010b). *Nursing's social policy statement: The essence of the profession.* Silver Spring, MD: Nursesbooks.org.

American Nurses Credentialing Center (ANCC). (2011a). ANCC nurse certification. Retrieved from http://www.nursecredentialing.org/Certification.aspx

American Nurses Credentialing Center (ANCC). (2011b). 2011 ANCC certification renewal. Retrieved from http://nursecredentialing.org/Certification/CertificationRenewal/RenewalofCertification.aspx

Brooten, D., Youngblut, J. M., Brown, L., Finkler, S. A., Neff, D. F., & Madigan, E. (2001). A randomized trial of nurse specialist home care for women with high-risk pregnancies: Outcomes and costs. *American Journal of Managed Care, 7*(8), 793–803.

Brooten, D., Youngblut, J. M., Kutcher, J., & Bobo, C. (2004). Quality and the nursing workforce: APNs, patient outcomes, and health care costs. *Nursing Outlook, 52*(1), 45–52.

Burns, N., & Grove, S. K. (2009). *The practice of nursing research: Appraisal, synthesis, and generation of evidence* (6th ed.). St. Louis: Elsevier, Saunders.

Creasia, J. L., & Reid, K. B. (2011). Pathways in nursing education. In J. L. Creasia and E. E. Friberg (Eds.), *Conceptual foundations: The bridge to professional nursing practice* (5th ed.). St. Louis: Elsevier, Mosby.

Gannett Healthcare Group. (2011). Nursing continuing education requirements by state. Retrieved from http://ce.nurse.com/RStateReqmnt.aspx/

Institute of Medicine (IOM). (2011). The future of nursing: Leading change, advancing health. Washington, DC: National Academies Press.

Kalb, K. B., Cherry, N. M., Kauzloric, J., Brender, A., Green, K., Miyagawa, L., & Shinoda-Mettler, A. (2006). A competency-based approach to public health nursing performance appraisal. *Public Health Nursing, 23*(2), 115–138.

Kutney-Lee, A., & Aiken, L. H. (2008). Effect of nurse staffing and education on the outcomes of surgical patients with co-morbid serious mental illness. *Psychiatric Services, 59*(12), 1466–1469.

Long, K. A. (2004). RN education: A matter of degrees. *Nursing, 34*(3), 48–49.

McMullan, M., Endacott, R., Gray M. A., Jasper, M., Miller, C. M. L., Scholes, J., & Webb, C. (2003). Portfolios and assessment of competence: A review of the literature. *Journal of Advanced Nursing, 41*(3), 283–294.

Melnyk, B. M., & Fineout-Overholt, E. (2005). *Evidence-based practice in nursing and healthcare: A guide to best practice.* Philadelphia, PA: Lippincott Williams & Wilkins.

Niebuhr, B., & Biel, M. (2007). The value of specialty nursing certification. *Nursing Outlook, 55*(4), 176–181.

Oermann, M. H. (2002). Developing a professional portfolio. *Orthopaedic Nursing, 21*(2), 73–78.

Ousley, A. L., Swarz, J. A., Milliken, E. L., & Ellis, S. (2010). Cancer education and effective dissemination: Information access is not enough. *Journal of Cancer Education, 25*(2), 196–205.

Quad Council of Public Health Nursing Organizations. (2004). Public health nursing competencies. *Public Health Nursing, 21*(5), 443–452.

Risjord, M. W. (2010). *Nursing knowledge: Science, practice, and philosophy.* Chichester, West Sussex, UK: Wiley-Blackwell.

Schweitzer, D. J., & Krassa, T. J. (2010). Deterrents to nurses' participation in continuing professional development: An integrative literature review. *Journal of Continuing Education in Nursing, 41*(10), 441–447.

Smith, K. N., Gunzenhauser, J. D., & Fielding, J. E. (2010). Reinvigorating performance evaluation: First steps in a local health department. *Public Health Nursing, 27*(5), 425–432.

Styles, M. M., Schumann, M. J., Bickford, C., & White, K. W. (2008). *Specialization and credentialing in nursing revisited: Understanding the issues, advancing the profession.* Silver Spring, MD: Nursesbooks.org.

CHAPTER 12

Standard 9. Evidence-Based Practice and Research

Kathleen M. White, PhD, RN, NEA-BC, FAAN

Standard 9. Evidence-Based Practice and Research. **The registered nurse integrates evidence and research findings into practice.**

Definition and Explanation of the Standard

Evidence-based practice (EBP) is the deliberate use of "a problem-solving approach to clinical decision-making within a healthcare organization that integrates the best available scientific evidence with the best available experiential (patient and practitioner) evidence, considers internal and external influences on practice, and encourages critical thinking in the judicious application of such evidence to the care of the individual patient, patient population or system" (Newhouse, Dearholt, Poe, Pugh, & White, 2007). EBP is an approach that enables clinicians to provide the highest quality of care to meet the multifaceted needs of their patients and families by using high-quality evidence to inform decision-making in their nursing practice (Melnyk & Fineout-Overholt, 2005).

EBP uses explicit methods to critically appraise and rate both the level (strength) and quality of evidence to answer a practice issue or question. In addition, to build an EBP, nurses use specific methods for incorporating evidence into practice as they consider the level of evidence and the implications for incorporating that evidence into the environmental context of care. The implications consider local practitioner expertise and practice patterns, organizational culture and experience data, and specific patients' preferences and values.

The EBP movement began in the 1970s when Archie Cochrane, a British epidemiologist, criticized his own profession for failing to implement the latest research into practice. The term *evidence-based medicine* was first used at the McMaster Medical School in Canada. In 1992, the Cochrane Collaboration was developed to synthesize available current clinical research to make it easier for clinicians to evaluate evidence for use in their practice. As the EBP movement became more widely adopted, it moved health care from a more traditional "do something or anything" focus to one of questioning clinicians' practice. Nursing began focusing on EBP strategies with the work of Stetler et al. (1998) and Titler et al. (2001).

However, even with the current emphasis on EBP for nursing, many nurses still continue to rely on outdated knowledge and traditions that they acquired as nursing students. Parahoo (2000) found that nurses lack confidence in their skills to evaluate the quality of research and lack confidence to implement change in the practice setting. Pravikoff, Tanner, and Pierce (2005) found that 61% of nurses need to seek information at least one time a week, but found that 67% of those nurses always or frequently sought information from a colleague instead of a reference text. Leasure, Stirlen, and Thompson (2008) surveyed nurse executives to identify the presence or absence of provider and organizational variables associated with use of EBP among nurses. The facilitators included staff members who read journals that publish original research and who participate in a journal club. Specific supportive infrastructure from the organization included the presence of a nursing research committee and a facility research committee as well as facility access to the Internet. The barriers to EBP were lack of staff involvement in projects, absence of communication about completed projects, and lack of knowledge about project outcomes. Among the respondents, 34% did not know what literature-searching capabilities were available to them in their facility.

Grounding nursing practice in evidence, rather than tradition, is necessary to meet nursing's social obligation of accountability to use current evidence-based nursing knowledge—including research findings—to guide their practice. Registered nurses are educated to evaluate and incorporate evidence into practice; to initiate appropriate changes to their practice on the basis of evidence; and to participate, as appropriate to their education level and position, in developing evidence through research. The graduate-level prepared specialty nurse or the advanced practice registered nurse (APRN) promotes a culture of clinical inquiry during clinical rounds and through mentoring of other nurses. Staff development, external presentations, and publications are important vehicles of communication of research results or EBP project synthesis. Both levels of nurses have the obligation to disseminate EBP findings to their peers and other health professionals. Improvement of outcomes is the goal of evidence-based practice.

Application of the Standard in Practice

Education

EBP must be an integrated part of nursing education programs. At the undergraduate level, the development and expansion of traditional research courses to include information and practice on searching and appraising research evidence is vital. Rather than isolating the teaching of EBP skills and knowledge to a sole research course, critical appraisal of evidence should also be integrated into every classroom and clinical learning experience. For example, while in the clinical setting, the instructor and students could choose a clinical procedure related to the clinical specialty and could search the evidence to evaluate whether the clinical facility's procedure is current and evidence-based. As a result of those kinds of experiences, the nurse of the future would approach every clinical situation with a critical appraisal of the evidence for clinical decision-making.

At the master's and doctoral level of education, students should expect to critically evaluate all aspects of practice (clinical, administrative, and education) and should expect this evaluation to be developed as an integrated thread throughout the curriculum. An expected outcome for students achieving this level of education is leading teams to facilitate EBP initiatives, including the dissemination of knowledge derived from the search and synthesis of evidence.

Involving a clinical librarian in the infusion and integration of EBP skills and knowledge across the curriculum is important. The librarian can be invaluable as a guest speaker to provide information on techniques for searching the evidence and on course-specific web sites and online resources that include high-quality sources of evidence-based materials. Introducing the librarian to the students should just be the start of their relationship. Many librarians now meet individually with students at all levels to help them answer clinical questions by searching the evidence.

Interprofessional education is a challenge and a tremendous opportunity to facilitate evidence-based practice. Nursing, medical, pharmacy, social work, physical therapy, and other allied health professional students, along with medical interns and residents in training, should participate in evaluating a common patient problem by searching and appraising the evidence together. In this way, they have the opportunity to discuss the relevant research findings and other clinical considerations, such as fit, feasibility, and appropriateness, for implementing the evidence into their specific practice.

Finally, developing the faculty's skills in evidence search techniques, critical appraisal, and the application of research evidence into practice is also an important consideration for nurse educators. As the educators develop their own skills in EBP techniques, they must incorporate the skills into their educational practices as they use evidence-based teaching techniques and as they model the need for evidence to drive their educational practice.

Administration

Administrative and organizational support is critical to establish a culture for EBP. Nurse administrators must consider the development and maintenance of EBP to be a strategic initiative and to provide adequate resources in the form of time, personnel, and money to develop EBP. Parahoo (2000) noted lack of leadership, vision, interest, motivation, strategy, and direction among managers to be huge barriers to developing an EBP. The EBP must be viewed as a critical element to the department of nursing's contribution to organizational goals and to meeting the organization's mission and vision.

To meet that mandate, nursing leadership must support EBP across the work continuum, including the development of job descriptions, orientation programs, and performance evaluations that support EBP as an expected competency. Nursing leadership must provide the staff with the time to develop and maintain EBP skills and knowledge. The leadership team should consider having mentors to facilitate the develop a strong foundation for EBP. The graduate-level specialty nurse and APRNs in the organization are an excellent example of a group that can be used to mentor and develop critical EBP skills and knowledge for staff nurses. The organization's committee structure is another way to develop and broadly infuse EBP skills and knowledge throughout the organization. A nurse researcher to mentor and guide nurses in their quests for an EBP can be hired directly or can be acquired through a collaboration with a school of nursing for the researcher's time. This nurse educator and researcher can participate in the unit's interprofessional rounds and collaborations, can facilitate journal clubs, and can guide the development of research projects.

To support EBP, administrators must require ongoing evaluation and documentation that nursing department policies and procedures are evidence-based. A clinical librarian can help the staff with this work. Additionally, staff nurses need to be supported to question their practice and have the autonomy to seek answers to practice issues and questions. Time is an important factor in EBP. The nurses must have tools available to them at the point of care, which means that computers with access to the Internet and online resources must be provided and available to all staff nurses in the clinical setting. Nurses must have access to databases, medication information, clinical practice guidelines, and decision support systems. See the Online Resources section in this chapter.

The PARIHS (Promoting Action on Research Implementation in Health Services) framework identifies three key elements to the translation of evidence to practice (Kitson et al., 2008). Two of those elements, context and facilitation, directly relate to the nurse administrator's responsibility in the implementation of EBP. It is important that the nursing leadership team also serve as role models for the use of EBP and to routinely search, evaluate, and base administrative and financial decisions on the best available evidence.

Performance and Quality Improvement

There is an increasing awareness of the importance of interprofessional collaboration to help the healthcare team deliver services effectively. The Institute of Medicine (2001) report titled *Crossing the Quality Chasm: A New Health System for the 21st Century* identified six aims for improvement in health care. One of those aims, effectiveness, specifically refers to providing services on the basis of scientific knowledge to all who would benefit from that service and to avoiding underuse and overuse of services for those who are unlikely to benefit from the service. Quality improvement efforts focus on systems and processes to identify and improve outcomes for all health professionals. Accessing, evaluating, and understanding the best available evidence for nursing practice is at the intersection of EBP and quality improvement processes. If the evidence for a practice change is conflicting or sufficiently lacking in quantity, a quality improvement evaluation of the evidence may be an important path to solving the practice issue or question.

Research

When nurses search for evidence to answer an EBP question and little or no evidence is found, a pilot study or full research project will be the only avenue to follow to answer the question. As discussed, a graduate-level specialty nurse, an APRN, a nurse educator, or a nurse researcher can mentor those conducting the research study. Interprofessional collaboration will make the research stronger and will increase the likelihood that a satisfactory practice change can eventually be implemented. When one is conducting research and quality improvement studies to evaluate a practice issue or question, attention to the organization's Institutional Review Board policies governing research on human subjects should be carefully examined and followed.

Conclusion

With the 2010 revision of the Standards of Professional Nursing Practice, the focus of the previous research standard was expanded and renamed Evidence-Based Practice and Research. The standard holds all registered nurses accountable to use evidence and research findings to guide their practice and to evaluate new evidence and research for practice changes.

Case Study and Discussion Topics

Case Study

The Standards of Care Committee is charged with reviewing Department of Nursing policies and procedures annually for currency and accuracy with new science. The policy on "Post-Operative Vital Signs" was due to be reviewed. The Post-Anesthesia Care Unit (PACU) and Medical–Surgical Unit educators collaborated to review the evidence for the current policy. They had difficulty finding readily available resources to inform the policy review. They decided to do a literature search and synthesis to establish an evidence-based policy on vital sign frequency in the post-operative period. They used the PICOT system to develop their question to frame the evidence search:

> **P** – (Patient, Population, or Problem): For adult hospitalized post-operative surgical patients.
>
> **I** – (Intervention): What frequency of vital signs.
>
> **C** – (Comparison with other treatments, if applicable): Not applicable.
>
> **O** – (Outcomes): Provision of the best monitoring safety for identifying complications.
>
> **T** – (Time): In the immediate post-operative period (24 hours).

The practice question was: For adult hospitalized patients, what frequency of vital signs during the immediate post-operative period provides the best monitoring safety for post-operative surgical patients on a medical–surgical unit in order to identify complications?

The educators searched the evidence. Then they identified, critiqued, and synthesized the evidence including one randomized controlled trial, three systematic reviews (at level III), five non-experimental studies, two national evidence-based guidelines, and two expert opinions were identified, critiqued, and synthesized. (See the summary in the following table.)

Johns Hopkins Nursing Evidence-Based Practice Model Synthesis and Recommendations Tool (Dearholt & Dang, 2012)			
Strength of Evidence	**Pieces of Evidence**	**Summary of Recommendations**	**Quality**
Level I Experimental (randomized controlled trial; [RCT]) or meta-analysis of RCTs	1	Fernandez (2005)	
Level II Quasi-experimental			
Level III Non-experimental or qualitative	8	Zeitz and McCutcheon (2002, 2006)—Vital signs are collected on the basis of tradition and are collected routinely, and there may not be a relationship between vital signs collection and the occurrence or detection of complications. The majority of clinical events occurred within the first 8 hours. The most common pattern of post-operative vital-signs collection (27%) is every hour for 4 hours and then every 4 hours for 4 times. The next most common (10%) was every 30 minutes for 2 hours, once an hour for 4 hours, and then every 4 hours. Zeitz (2003); Evans (2001)—Both are systematic reviews. Post-operative vital signs are collected routinely and are based on tradition, not on individual patient need or evidence. Systematic Review (2004)—There is limited information regarding the frequency with which vital signs should be monitored, much of which is based on surveys of nurses, clinical practice reports, and expert opinion. Two studies (1990, 1995) recommended this: every 15 minutes × 1; every 30 minutes × 2; every 60 minutes × 1; and every 4 hours × 4.	B

(Continued)

Johns Hopkins Nursing Evidence-Based Practice Model Synthesis and Recommendations Tool (Dearholt & Dang, 2012) (*Continued*)			
Strength of Evidence	**Pieces of Evidence**	**Summary of Recommendations**	**Quality**
Level IV Opinion of nationally recognized experts, which is based on research evidence	2	The American Society of PeriAnesthesia Nurses' 2006–2008 Standards of Perianesthesia Nursing Practice does not specify how frequently vital signs need to be taken. Frequency is patient-specific according to stability of condition and degree of variance from baseline. Most institutions have a policy to take vital signs every 5 minutes for the first 15 minutes, and then every 10 to 15 minutes for the duration of the stay depending on patient stability and return to baseline. If the patient is very unstable, perhaps on vasoactive drips, the frequency will be at least every 5 minutes until the patient is more stable. It is unusual to find a time span greater than 15 minutes in Phase I PACU unless the patient is a boarder or awaiting transfer to another area.	
Level V Opinion of nationally recognized experts, which is based on nonresearch evidence	2	Post-operative vital signs are collected routinely, are based on tradition, and are not based on individual patient need or evidence.	B–C

(*Note:* All sources cited in this table are from Dearholt & Drang, 2012.)

Conclusion: No clear evidence exists to change policy; however, several suggestions could be made:

- Define time frames for vital sign monitoring in the immediate post-operative period.

- Define vital signs.

- Describe what level of personnel should monitor the vital signs.

Discussion Topics

- How should the earlier suggestions be accomplished?

- What should the educators now do in accordance with the EBP project recommendation?

- How should staff nurses be involved in seeking additional information?

- How can this type of work in nursing be accomplished routinely?

Online Resources

Cumulative Index to Nursing and Allied Health Literature (CINAHL®)

The database for publications in the fields of nursing and allied health from 1982 through the present includes more than 1,500 nursing and allied health journal titles and more than 700,000 citations. The CINAHL Subject Headings are nursing and allied health terms and include nursing classifications. CINAHL has evidence-based filters and systematic review and meta-analysis as subject headings. Access CINAHL online at http://www.ebscohost.com/academic/cinahl-plus-with-full-text/

Cochrane Library

The library provides access to information compiled by the Cochrane Collaboration, an international network that maintains and disseminates a collection of seven evidence-based databases about the effects of interventions in health care. Access the Cochrane Library online at www.cochrane.org

Database of Abstracts of Reviews of Effects (DARE)

The database is maintained by the Centre for Reviews and Dissemination, University of York, as part of the United Kingdom's National Institute for Health Research. DARE contains 15,000 abstracts of systematic reviews, including more than 6,000 quality-assessed reviews and details of all Cochrane reviews and protocols. The database focuses on the effects of interventions used in health and social care. It is updated weekly and may include reviews that have not yet been added to the Cochrane Library. Access DARE online at http://www.crd.york.ac.uk/CMS2Web/

Google Scholar

This site applies Google search methodology on the basis of key words. It sorts articles weighing full text, author, publication, and the number of citations. Access Google Scholar online at http://scholar.google.com

Joanna Briggs Institute (JBI)

Established in 1996 by University of Adelaide and Royal Adelaide Hospital to facilitate evidence-based practice, JBI promotes the synthesis, transfer, and use of evidence through identifying feasible, appropriate, meaningful, and effective healthcare practices to assist in the improvement of healthcare outcomes globally. It includes 25 collaborating centers in 40 countries. The JBI web site includes evidence in the form of a systematic review or evidence synthesis on clinical questions. Access JBI online at www.joannabriggs.edu.au

National Guideline Clearinghouse (NGC)

The NGC is a resource for evidence-based clinical practice guidelines. It is maintained by the Agency for Healthcare Research and Quality (AHRQ) and the U.S. Department of Health and Human Services. Access NGC online at either www.ahrq.gov or www.guideline.gov

PubMed/MEDLINE

This site is the primary database of information in medical and health sciences fields, including the International Nursing Index, a subset of MEDLINE. It is produced by the U.S. National Library of Medicine and covers journals from 1966 through the present. There are more than 4,600 biomedical, nursing, and dental journal titles and more than 17 million citations. PubMed uses MeSH (Medical Subject Headings) for indexing. It uses evidence-based filters for clinical queries, systematic reviews, and practice guidelines and can use the limit function to look specifically for meta-analyses. Access PubMed online at http://www.ncbi.nlm.nih.gov/pubmed/

Trip Database—Clinical Search Engine (Trip)

The Trip Database was created in 1997 in the United Kingdom as a clinical search tool designed to allow health professionals to rapidly identify the highest-quality clinical evidence for clinical practice. Access the Trip Database online at www.tripdatabase.com

SUMSearch

SUMSearch does real-time meta-searches of high-quality medical web sites. It combines meta-searching and contingency searching in order to automate searching for medical evidence. Access SUMSearch online at http://library. uthscsa.edu/2011/10/sumsearch/

Virginia Henderson International Nursing Library (VHINL) Database

This database includes the Registry of Nursing Research sponsored by Sigma Theta Tau International, which is the International Honor Society of Nursing. It includes open access to *Worldviews on Evidence-Based Nursing*, a collection of evidence and literature reviews. Access VHINL online at http://www. nursinglibrary.org/vhl/

References and Other Sources

Dearholt, S., White, K., Newhouse, R., Poe, S., & Pugh, L. (2008). Making the vision a reality: Educational strategies to develop evidence-based practice mentors. *Journal of Nurses in Staff Development, 24*(2), 1–7.

Dearholt, S., and Dang, D., eds (2012). *Johns Hopkins Nursing Evidence-Based Practice: Model and Guidelines* 2nd edition. Indianapolis, IN: Sigma Theta Tau International.

Institute of Medicine. (IOM) (2001). *Crossing the quality chasm: A new health system for the 21st century.* Washington, DC: National Academies Press.

Kitson, A., Rycroft-Malone, J., Harvey, G., McCormack, B., Seers, K., & Titchen, A. (2008). Evaluating the successful implementation of evidence into practice using the PARIHS framework: Theoretical and practical challenges. *Implementation Science, 3*(1). doi:10.1186/1748-5908-3-1

Leasure, A. R., Stirlen, J., & Thompson, C. (2008). Barriers and facilitators to the use of evidence-based best practices. *Dimensions of Critical Care Nursing, 27*(2), 74–84.

Melnyk, B. M., & Fineout-Overholt, E. (2005). *Evidence-based practice in nursing and healthcare: A guide to best practice.* Philadelphia, PA: Lippincott Williams & Wilkins.

Newhouse, R., Dearholt, S., Poe, S., Pugh, L., & White, K. (2007). *Johns Hopkins nursing evidence-based practice model and guidelines.* Indianapolis, IN: Sigma Theta Tau International.

Parahoo, K. (2000). Barriers to, and facilitators of, research utilization among nurses in Northern Ireland. *Journal of Advanced Nursing, 31,* 89–98.

Pravikoff, D., Tanner, A., & Pierce, S. (2005). Readiness of U.S. nurses for evidence-based practice: Many don't understand or value research and have had little or no training to help them find evidence on which to base their practice. *American Journal of Nursing, 105*(9), 40–51.

Stetler, C., Brunell, M., Giulano, K., Morsi, D., Prince, L., & Newell-Stokes, V. (1998). Evidence-based practice and the role of nursing leadership. *Journal of Nursing Administration, 28*(7/8), 45–53.

Titler, M. G., Kleiber, C., Steelman, V. J., Rakel, B. A., Budreau, G., Everett, L. Q., et al. (2001). The Iowa Model of evidence-based practice to promote quality care. *Critical Care Nursing Clinics of North America, 13*(4), 497–509.

CHAPTER 13

Standard 10. Quality of Practice

Brenda L. Lyon, PhD, CNS, FAAN

Standard 10. Quality of Practice. **The registered nurse contributes to quality nursing practice.**

Definition and Explanation of the Standard

The registered nurse (RN) contributes to quality nursing practice by assuring that patients receive evidence-based care that is patient-centered, safe, effective, timely, efficient, and equitable (IOM, 2001). The word *quality* has many usages in health care, both as an adjective and a noun, but those uses are grounded in the dictionary sense of the word: a peculiar or essential character, a degree of excellence, or a distinguishing attribute (Merriam-Webster, 2012). The following definition from the current edition of *Nursing: Scope and Standards of Practice* (ANA, 2010, p. 67) is nurse-sensitive:

> *Quality.* The degree to which health services for patients, families, groups, communities, or populations increase the likelihood of desired outcomes and are consistent with current professional knowledge.

Nurses at all levels have a pivotal role in quality health care. The Institute of Medicine (IOM) report, *Keeping Patients Safe: Transforming the Work Environment of Nurses* (IOM, 2004), makes recommendations for healthcare organizations to improve the quality of care in hospitals, nursing homes, and other healthcare organization work environments that threaten patient safety through their effect on nursing care.

The IOM (2003, 2011) identified core competencies necessary for all healthcare professionals, regardless of discipline, to ensure quality healthcare outcomes. Those competencies include knowledge and skills in the following:

- Provide patient-centered care that encompasses the uniqueness of each patient.

- Work on interdisciplinary teams to integrate care, thereby ensuring that care is continuous and reliable.

- Use evidence-based practice that integrates research evidence with clinical expertise and patient preference.

- Apply quality improvement principles and strategies to change patient care processes and systems of care.

- Use informatics to communicate and support decision-making to reduce errors.

Quality is everyone's responsibility in health care; however, Standard 10 identifies the nurses' responsibility in ensuring quality of care. Because of their clinical expertise and direct position at the point of care with health-care consumers, nurses have individual responsibility and accountability for quality care. Those contributions to ensuring quality care occur directly through clinical practice activities as well as indirectly through the practice environment when quality care is made a priority. Nurses have embraced this priority and have traditionally been involved in interprofessional quality improvement efforts. Nurses have provided care that meets appropriate standards and have been involved in continuous quality improvement to improve nursing services and health care for their patients. Nurses are engaged every day in identifying areas for improvement, for monitoring, for measuring, and for reporting quality.

Quality nursing care is essential to cost-effective patient care that achieves desired outcomes (Lee et al., 1999; Aiken, 2008). The advanced practice registered nurse (APRN) contributes to quality nursing practice by leading the design and implementation of quality improvements in patient care processes and procedures, by designing and evaluating innovations in practice to improve health outcomes, by bringing research evidence to the point of care, by generating research questions pertinent to quality healthcare outcomes, and by leading healthcare system changes targeting the improvement of care. As part of the larger interprofessional team, nurses at all levels of practice formulate recommendations for improvement and design innovations, and they sustain improvements in quality and safety to enhance healthcare delivery and nursing practice.

Through quality improvement efforts, nurses—as the key caregivers in hospitals—significantly influence the quality of care provided and, ultimately, the effectiveness of treatment and patient outcomes. To be eligible for Magnet® designation, hospital organizations must promote quality that supports a professional practice environment and that encourages nurses to express concerns about the practice environment. Moreover, a Magnet organization must lead initiatives to improve the practice environment.

Application of the Standard to Practice

Education

Educators design curricula that help nursing students acquire the competencies required to contribute to quality nursing care. To that end, students attain the requisite knowledge about nursing's unique contribution to patient care. They do so through a systematic approach to nursing care using the nursing process. Nursing students learn to accurately assess and diagnose patient problems amenable to and requiring nursing intervention and therapeutics. To do so, they learn the identification of etiologies that determine the nursing interventions needed (Lyon, 2009) so that they achieve the desired nurse-sensitive outcomes (Doran, 2010). Learning experiences are structured so that students recognize the importance of evidence-based care and tracking of the quality indicators of nursing care as explicated in the American Nurses Association's National Database of Nursing Quality Indicators® (NDNQI®, 2011). Students also become knowledgeable about other policy groups such as The Joint Commission (2011), Agency for Healthcare Research and Quality (AHRQ, 2011), Institute for Healthcare Improvement (IHI, 2011), and National Quality Forum (2011), all of which influence the national standards for quality patient outcomes.

Staff development educators focus on creating opportunities for staff members to maintain knowledge and skill competencies in the context of complex multidisciplinary systems and to acquire new knowledge and skill competencies to effectively run and monitor new technology. APRNs work with staff nurses to advance those nurses' knowledge in reading and critiquing research so they can identify new knowledge appropriately applicable to the practice setting. Additionally, APRNs mentor staff members in bridging the gap between what is learned through research and the care that is provided to patients. Bridging the gap is also captured by developing and evaluating evidence-based policies, procedures, and guidelines to improve the quality of practice and the practice environment to achieve desired patient outcomes.

The RN must recognize and value the important contributions of nursing care to patient outcomes because self-determination is largely affected by values. Values are imperatives for action. When the RN values the work of nursing for its contribution to quality outcomes, then the RN, with a self-determined priority, maintains competency and continues to advance knowledge and skills.

Administration

The culture of a healthcare institution can affect safety and quality outcomes (Richardson & Storr, 2010). Therefore, administrators ensure that the standard is accomplished by developing policies and procedures, standards of practice, job descriptions, performance appraisals, and expectations for individual development plans for the organization. Those plans are consistent with the expectation that RNs should contribute to quality nursing practice. It is important for administrators to have a leadership style that fosters a healthy work environment in which nurses have autonomy along with self-governance and where nurses who are inquisitive and speak up about patient quality and safety are respected and appreciated (Mardon, Khanna, Sorra, Dyer, & Famolaro, 2010; Adams, Erickson, Ives, Jones, & Paulo, 2009; Cummings, Midodzi, Wong, & Estabrooks, 2010).

Performance and Quality Improvement

In today's regulatory environment, healthcare institutions must be continuously focused on quality assurance and improvement. Most institutions have staff members devoting 100% of their time in this area. Examples of quality improvement initiatives are the reduction of nosocomial infections such as ventilator-associated pneumonia, elimination of central-line infections, and elimination of urinary tract infections (Kanouff, DeHaven, & Kaplan, 2008). Additionally, it is important that RNs participate in quality improvement activities with an ongoing spirit of inquiry whereby they identify areas of concern when something is or is not happening in terms of patient outcomes. Also, RNs need to actively participate in quality improvement projects by documenting and tracking outcomes. Additionally, managers, quality improvement staff members, and APRNs lead quality improvement efforts and provide feedback to the interprofessional team about progress in achieving and maintaining nurse-sensitive outcomes (Albanese et al., 2010).

Research

Research for nursing practice is essential because it generates new knowledge about the effectiveness of nursing care, and it encourages clinical inquiry investigations that identify opportunities for quality improvement or that evaluate interventions designed to improve patient outcomes. RNs contribute to research by asking important clinical questions pertinent to the effectiveness of nursing care and patient outcomes and by sharing those questions with APRNs and nurse researchers. Examples of important clinical questions that have resulted in research informing the practice of nursing and improving patient outcomes include the following:

1. What patient- and environment-related factors contribute to patient falls (Murphy, Labonte, Klock, & Houser, 2008)?

2. What patient- and nursing care-related factors contribute to the development of pressure ulcers (Wound, Ostomy, and Continence Nurses Society, 2003)?

3. What patient- and nursing care-related factors contribute to ventilator-acquired pneumonia (VAP) (Vollman, 2006)?

Conclusion

Improving healthcare quality and patient safety is a high priority on the national healthcare agenda, and nurses are integral to the healthcare system's efforts to improve quality. As healthcare organizations, large and small, participate in a wide range of quality improvement activities, they rely on nurses to help address those demands. Nurses are critical to such activities because of their day-to-day patient care responsibilities. For the well-being of patients and the cost-effectiveness of care, RNs, APRNs, and all graduate specialty nurses must practice in a manner consistent with the Quality of Practice standard. Nurses who are committed to quality practice make important contributions to quality improvement efforts in healthcare institutions and to research focused on improving patient outcomes.

Case Study and Discussion Topics

Case Study

You are a critical-care staff and clinical nurse working at Eminent Hospital in Trustworthy, Kansas. The hospital is a 320-bed acute-care facility. You work the day 12-hour shift rotation on Thursdays, Fridays, and Saturdays on a 24-bed Intensive Care Unit. Typical length of stay on the unit is 5–7 days, and many patients are on ventilators. The VAP rate has been effectively reduced to 0 by staff members, who have diligently followed the VAP-prevention protocol over the past 6 months. The VAP initiative was kicked off 7 months ago by unit staff members in collaboration with their Clinical Nurse Specialist (CNS). However, today (Thursday), the staff members received a report from their CNS that the unit had four patients who developed early-stage decubiti over the past 2 weeks. Previously, the unit had been running an incidence rate of less than one per month.

Discussion Topics

Respond to the following questions:

1. What patient assessment data need to be collected for this case?

2. Identify nursing care and environmental factors that might be contributing to the development of decubiti. What data need to be collected and examined to help with the determination and validation of each possible contributing factor?

3. What nursing care interventions would be required to effectively alter the factors and etiologies that you have identified?

4. Discuss the role of the RN and APRN in quality improvement.

References and Other Sources

Adams, J. M., Erickson, J. I., Ives, J., Jones, D. A., & Paulo, L. (2009). An evidence-based structure for transformative nurse executive practice: The model of interrelationship of leadership, environments, and outcomes for nurse executives (MILE ONE). *Nursing Administration Quarterly, 33*(4), 280–287.

Agency for Healthcare Research and Quality (AHRQ). (2011). Retrieved from http://www. ahrq.gov

Aiken, L. H. (2008). Economics of nursing. *Policy, Politics, and Nursing Practice, 9*(2), 73–79.

Albanese, M. P., Evans, D. A., Schantz, C. A., Bowen, M., Moffa, J. S., Piesieski, P., & Polomano, R. C. (2010). Engaging clinical nurses in quality and performance improvement activities. *Nursing Administration Quarterly, 34*(3), 226–245.

American Nurses Association (ANA). (2010). *Nursing: Scope and standards of practice* (2nd ed.). Silver Spring, MD: Nursesbooks.org.

Cummings, G. G., Midodzi, W. K., Wong, C. A., & Estabrooks, C. A. (2010). The contribution of hospital nursing leadership styles to 30-day patient mortality. *Nursing Research, 59*(5), 331–339.

Doran, D. M. (2010). *Nursing outcomes: State of the science* (2nd ed.). Sudbury, MA: Jones & Bartlett Publishers.

Institute for Healthcare Improvement (IHI). (2011). Retrieved from http://www.ihi.org

Institute of Medicine (IOM). (2001). *Crossing the quality chasm: A new health system for the 21st century.* Washington, DC: National Academies Press.

Institute of Medicine (IOM). (2003). *Health professions education: A bridge to quality.* Washington, DC: National Academies Press.

Institute of Medicine (IOM). (2004). *Keeping patients safe: Transforming the work environment of nurses.* Washington, DC: National Academies Press.

Institute of Medicine (IOM). (2011). *The future of nursing: Leading change, advancing health.* Washington, DC: National Academies Press.

The Joint Commission. (2011). Facts about the Joint Commission Center for Transforming Healthcare. Oakbrook Terrace, IL: Center for Transforming Healthcare. Retrieved from http://www.centerfortransforminghealthcare.org/about

Kanouff, A. J., DeHaven, K. D., & Kaplan, P. D. (2008) Prevention of nosocomial infections in the intensive care unit. *Critical Care Nursing Quarterly, 31*(4), 302–308.

Lee, J. L., Chang, B. L., Change, M. L., Pearson, K. L., Kahn, K. L., & Rubenstein, L. V. (1999). Does what nurses do affect clinical outcomes for hospitalized patients? A review of the literature. *Health Services Research, 34*(5), 1011–1032.

Lyon, B. L. (2009). A clinical reasoning model: A clinical inquiry guide for solving problems in the nursing domain. In J. Fulton, B. L. Lyon, & K. A. Goudreau (Eds.), *Foundations of clinical nurse specialist practice* (pp. 61–74). New York: Springer Publishing Co.

Mardon, R. E., Khanna, K., Sorra, J., Dyer, N., & Famolaro, T. (2010). Exploring relationships between hospital patient safety culture and adverse events. *Journal of Patient Safety, 6*(4), 226–232.

Merriam-Webster. (2012). *Online dictionary.* http://www.merriam-webster.com/dictionary/quality

Murphy, T. H., Labonte, P., Klock, M., & Houser, L. (2008). Falls prevention for elders in acute care: An evidence-based nursing practice initiative. *Critical Care Nursing Quarterly, 31*(1), 33–39.

National Database of Nursing Quality Indicators® (NDNQI®). (2011). Retrieved from http://www.nursingquality.org

National Quality Forum. (2011). Retrieved from http://www.qualityforum.org

Richardson, A., & Storr, J. (2010). Patient safety: A literature review on the impact of nursing empowerment, leadership and collaboration. *International Nursing Review, 57*(1), 12–21.

Wound, Ostomy, and Continence Nurses Society. (2003). *Guideline for prevention and management of pressure ulcers.* Mt. Laurel, NJ: Author.

Vollman, K. M. (2006). Ventilator-associated pneumonia and pressure ulcer prevention as targets for quality improvement in the ICU. *Critical Care Nursing Clinics of North America, 18*(4), 453–467.

CHAPTER 14

Standard 11. Communication

Ann O'Sullivan, MS, RN, CNE, NE-BC

Standard 11. Communication. **The registered nurse communicates effectively in a variety of formats in all areas of practice.**

Definition and Explanation of the Standard

Effective interpersonal communication (IPC) between nurses and the healthcare consumer is one of the most important elements for improving satisfaction, compliance, and health outcomes. Effective IPC is necessary to perform an assessment and to make an accurate diagnosis that is based on a full disclosure of information by the healthcare consumer, thus leading to an appropriate plan of care that the consumer can agree to. The nurse must ensure that the healthcare consumer understands his or her medical condition, as well as the rationale behind a treatment regimen.

Communication is a complex feedback loop that requires a sender, a message, and a receiver. The mode through which the message is sent and received can be verbal, nonverbal, spoken, or written. A key principle of effective communication is that the only true communication is what the other person perceives you to have said, written, or intended.

There are three communication styles. *Passive communication* is described as having the goal of avoiding conflict at all cost. The actual behavior is one of (1) ignoring one's own rights, being inhibited, not speaking up, or avoiding eye contact; (2) having a soft, weak, wavering voice; or (3) being vague, rambling, and apologetic. This style is not very effective because passive communicators do not meet their own needs, the unit does not benefit from their wisdom and contributions, and they often suffer from physical, mental, and emotional illnesses related to "keeping it all bottled up inside."

Aggressive communication is characterized as competitive, controlling, manipulative, dominating, bossy, loud, demanding, sarcastic, and blaming. The aggressive communicator's goal is to win regardless of the cost to others. This style is not effective because everyone loses in the long run. The senders may get what they want for a short time, but that satisfaction generally does not last. Others do not respect, follow, or comply with the sender's wishes for very long, if at all.

Assertive communication is described as adult communication with the goal of win–win. It is open, honest communication that results in respect of self and others. Characteristics consist of expressing oneself without violating the rights of others; remaining calm, confident, and relaxed; taking responsibility for one's own behavior; seeing and making choices; and being open to negotiation. This communication style is hard and needs to be learned through continued study and practice. People who routinely communicate in an assertive manner generally experience successful relationships in their marriages, workplaces, and professional and personal relationships.

When stress is added, perceptions get tangled. In general, the communication feedback loop works well when there is no stress. It is up to the sender and the receiver to communicate in such a way as to minimize the stress and to maximize the chance that the true intention is what is perceived and acted upon. This approach becomes especially challenging in today's fast-paced, emailing, texting, and technology-driven world.

Communication is a hot topic in health care today. The American Association of Colleges of Nursing (IPEC, 2011) identifies skilled communication as a core competency for interprofessional collaborative practice as follows: Communicate with patients, families, communities, and other health professionals in a responsive and responsible manner that supports a team approach to the maintenance of health and the treatment of disease. The Joint Commission suggests that ineffective communication is a top contributor to sentinel events. Intimidating and disruptive behaviors can foster medical errors; contribute to poor patient satisfaction and to preventable adverse outcomes; increase the cost of care; and cause qualified clinicians, administrators, and managers to seek new positions in more professional environments. The safety and quality of patient care depend on teamwork, communication, and a collaborative work environment (The Joint Commission, 2008).

Studies have indicated that more than 60% of medication errors were caused by mistakes in interpersonal communication (Maxfield, Grenney, McMillan, Patterson, & Switzer, 2005). Each year, hundreds of thousands of patients are harmed during their treatments because of fundamental problems in the collective behavior of the caring professionals who care for them (Kohn, Corrigan, Donaldson, 2000). Eastbaugh (2004, p. 36) reports, "The most common cause of malpractice suits is failed communicating with patients and their families."

In 2005, the American Association of Critical-Care Nurses (AACN) and VitalSmarts® conducted a nationwide study, *Silence Kills* (Maxfield et al., 2005), that suggested that people in health care frequently failed to have crucial conversations, which would likely add to unacceptable error rates. This study recommends that improvement in those crucial conversations will contribute to significant reductions in errors, improvement in quality of care, reduction in nursing turnover, and marked improvement in productivity. However, *fewer than 1 in 10 fully discussed their concerns with the other person.* And most do not believe they have the responsibility to bring their concerns to the attention of the other person. About half of the respondents say the concerns have lasted for more than a year. A significant number reported that there have been serious injurious consequences of the concerning behavior (Maxfield et al., 2005).

In the follow-up study, *Silent Treatment* (Maxfield, Grenny, Lavandero, & Groah, 2010), 58% of the nurses reported that they had been in situations where they felt unsafe to speak up about the problems or where they were unable to get others to listen. The nurses cited that their lack of ability to speak up, belief that it was not their job, and low confidence that speaking up would do any good were the three primary obstacles to direct communication. Other obstacles included time and fear of retaliation. The three main "undiscussables" were dangerous shortcuts, incompetence, and disrespect.

A discussion of communication is not complete without including today's new communication networks. Social networks and the Internet provide great opportunities for exchange and dissemination of knowledge among nurses. Online social networking can enhance collegial communication among nurses and can provide opportunities for continued professional education. At the same time, the social networks have great potential for violating patient confidentiality, damaging the public trust in healthcare providers, and damaging a nurse's professional and personal future. *ANA's Principles for Social Networking and the Nurse* (ANA, 2011a) offers essential principles for all nurses to follow:

- Nurses must not transmit or place online individually identifiable patient information.

- Nurses who interact with patients on social media must observe ethically prescribed professional boundaries.

- Nurses should evaluate all their postings with the understanding that a patient, colleague, educational institution, or employer could potentially view those postings.

- Nurses should take advantage of privacy settings available on many social network sites.

Application of the Standard in Practice

Many states have nurse practice acts that identify obligations for nurses related to providing for safe and effective nursing care, including communication that advocates for the healthcare consumer and communication and collaboration with other healthcare professionals.

Education

Nurse educators play a key role in teaching and modeling assertive, effective communication skills to students. Nursing curricula must include communication competencies in clinical and theory courses; classes in therapeutic communication with healthcare consumers; and effective, assertive communication for structured communication, conflict management, and negotiation among healthcare providers. Case studies and role-playing are effective tools for teaching students those skills.

Incivility is a term used to describe rude, disruptive, intimidating, and undesirable behaviors that are directed toward another person (Clark & Ahten, 2010). A faculty has a dual role in addressing the problem of incivility: (1) teach and model civil, respectful behavior to set expectations for students' professional behaviors and (2) identify the behaviors students should expect from others in the workplace. Students must learn to identify uncivil, unacceptable behaviors, especially the more subtle disruptive behaviors of eye-rolling, sarcastic comments, taunting, and other disrespectful ways of communicating. Faculty members have an important role in helping students identify and correct such behaviors in themselves and in teaching strategies to deal with this problem in others. The faculty must establish safe, engaging learning environments that will help to reduce student stress and anxiety. "In our experience, it is a 'short walk' from unresolved anxiety to incivility" (Clark & Ahten, 2010).

Administration

Nurse administrators are responsible for ensuring that behavioral standards, policies, and procedures related to effective communication are in place and enforced. Communication competencies should be a part of the performance evaluation tool. Healthy workplaces and cultures of safety and of open, honest communication are initiated at the administrative level and are essential components of patient safety and quality and of a professional work environment. The *Standards for a Healthy Work Environment* (AACN, 2005) includes a standard on communication: "Nurses must be as proficient in communication skills as they are in clinical skills." The administrator is responsible for creating and sustaining a work environment that fosters open and direct communication.

Disruptive behavior in the workplace is not new, but it is an issue that must be addressed by nurse managers and administrators in all settings. There are many names for this behavior: lateral violence, bullying, abuse, verbal violence, incivility, mobbing, and so forth. The result of this behavior is "The perpetrator physically, verbally, or emotionally abuses an employee and consequences may arise from this event" (CAN, 2008; p. 2). Prevalence of workplace violence is well reported in the literature and ranges from 53% to 86% (ANA, 2011b).

The ANA (2012) affirmed its stand on workplace violence with the following resolution, which stated the following:

- Nurses have the right to work in environments free from abusive behaviors.

- Nurses should respect the dignity of all individuals including colleagues through the maintenance of caring relationship.

- Nurses should report incidences of abuse.

- Nurses should advocate for policies to support violence-free workplaces.

Nurse administrators in all healthcare settings must use specific strategies to reduce disruptive communication patterns (see http://www.jointcommission.org), including the following examples:

- Educate all team members on appropriate, effective communication, and professional behavior (e.g., dealing with verbal violence and bullying, dealing with difficult patients, and using specific strategies for communicating in difficult situations).

- Hold team members accountable for interprofessional communication and handoffs.

- Develop and implement specific policies and processes related to verbal violence and bullying.

- Provide skill-based training and coaching for all leaders in management development on effective communication.

To improve communication and the work environment, SBAR (situation, background, assessment, recommendations) and ISBAR (includes identification as the first step) are strategies that have been developed to address this challenge in effective communication. Handoffs (verbal exchange of information between healthcare providers about a patient's condition, treatment plan, care needs, etc.) commonly occur at change of shift and when patients are transferred to other units or facilities. Using SBAR can help communicate vital information in an organized, comprehensive manner that will provide assurance of safe, quality care (Jordan, 2009). Research has shown that teaching this method of communication has improved communication outcomes among healthcare professionals (Marshall, Harrison, & Flanagan, 2009).

Performance and Quality Improvement

Specific competencies that are essential to meet the Communication standard are achieving self-assessment and continuous improvement of one's communication skills; questioning the rationale for care decisions when they do not appear to be in the patient's best interest; and contributing one's own professional perspective in discussions with the interprofessional team.

The Essential Guide to Nursing Practice

The Joint Commission issued Sentinel Event Alert 40 in 2008. It called for a new leadership standard to address disruptive and inappropriate behaviors and included these:

- The hospital or organization should have a code of conduct that defines acceptable and disruptive and inappropriate behaviors.

- Leaders should create and implement a process for managing disruptive and inappropriate behavior.

The previously noted studies—*Silence Kills* (Maxfield et al., 2005) and *Silent Treatment* (Maxfield et al., 2010)—also provide evidence that lack of communication causes problems with patient safety. Quality improvement initiatives must address communication failures in any patient safety problems or other process failures that occur in any setting. Root Cause Analysis and Failure Mode Effect Analysis are quality improvement methods that are vital to uncovering those communication failures.

Research

Nurse researchers need to participate in ongoing research to uncover the key communication issues in health care and strategies for improving communication in order to improve the quality of patient care. Also inherent in the nurse's role is the need to use research findings to resolve communication issues in practice. Funding for research in communication issues is often lacking. Ongoing research is needed on the effects of communication on patient safety and healthy work environments. Root cause analysis studies are essential processes in discovering what communication errors contribute to failures in patient safety.

Conclusion

Standard 11 states that the registered nurse communicates effectively in a variety of formats in all areas of practice. Research has shown that effective communication is essential to safe, quality patient care and to healthy work environments that lead to nurse satisfaction and staff retention. Nurse clinicians, educators, administrators, and researchers all have a vital role in providing assurance that patterns of communication promote safe patient care and healthy work environments.

Case Studies and Discussion Topics

1. A group of nurses on a medical surgical unit describe a peer as careless and inattentive. Instead of confronting her, they double-check her work—sometimes re-checking a critical patient's vital signs after she has done them. They've worked around this nurse's weaknesses for more than a year. They resent her, but never talk to her about their concerns.

   a. How does this behavior violate the communication standard and competencies?

   b. What is your role in dealing with this situation?

2. The nurse is trying to follow the time-out policy and to make sure the surgical site marking is done. The physician refuses to follow the procedure.

   a. How should the nurse deal with this physician situation?

   b. What communication competency is particularly relevant here?

3. A nurse educator observes staff nurses being disrespectful and making sarcastic comments about the first-year nursing students on the unit.

   a. How should the instructor deal with this issue?

   b. What and how should she teach the students about this example of incivility?

4. Mr. Jones is being discharged from the hospital with congestive heart failure.

   a. Today is the first time the nurse has cared for this patient. How should he or she assess the patient's and family's preference for receiving this discharge information? What factors would be particularly important to consider?

   b. How would the nurse assess his or her effectiveness in meeting the patient and family's discharge information needs?

References and Other Sources

American Association of Critical-Care Nurses (AACN). (2005). *AACN standards for establishing and maintaining healthy work environments.* Mission Viejo, CA: Author.

The Essential Guide to Nursing Practice

American Nurses Association (ANA). (2010). *Nursing: Scope and standards of practice* (2nd ed.). Silver Spring, MD: Nursesbooks.org.

American Nurses Association (ANA). (2011a). *ANA's principles for social networking and the nurses.* Silver Spring, MD: Author.

American Nurses Association (ANA). (2011b) *Workplace violence.* Retrieved from www.nursingworld.org/workplaceviolence

American Nurses Association (ANA). (2012). *Bullying in the workplace: Reversing a culture–2012 edition.* Silver Spring, MD: Author.

Center for the American Nurse (CAN). (2008). *Bullying in the workplace: Reversing a culture.* Silver Spring, MD: Author.

Clark, C., & Ahten, S. (2010). Beginning the conversation: The nurse educator's role in preventing incivility in the workplace. *RN Idaho, 33,* 9–10.

Eastaugh, S. (2004). Reducing litigation costs through better patient communication. *The Physician Executive. 30*(3), 36–38. Retrieved from http://net.acpe.org/membersonly/pejournal/2004/MayJune/Articles/ Eastbaugh_Steven.pdf

Georgia Department of Community Health's Health Care Workforce Policy Advisory Committee. (2002). *Promoting health care workplace excellence.* Retrieved from http://www.georgia.gov/vgn/images/portal/cit_1210/44/ 62/32488427wpac_2002.pdf

Hughes, N. (2009). Bullies in health care beware. *American Nurse Today, 3*(6), 35.

Interprofessional Education Collaborative Expert Panel (IPEC). (2011). *Core competencies for interprofessional collaborative practice: Report of an expert panel.* Washington, DC: Interprofessional Education Collaborative.

The Joint Commission. (2008, July 9). Behaviors that undermine a culture of safety. (Issue 40). Retrieved from http://www.jointcommission.org/ assets/1/18/SEA_40.PDF

Jordan, K. (2009, February 17). SBAR: A communication formula for patient safety. *Boston.com.* Retrieved from http://www.boston.com/jobs/ healthcare/oncall/articles/2009/02/17/perspective/

Kohn, L., Corrigan, J., & Donaldson, M., (Eds.). (2000). *To err is human: Building a safer health system.* Washington, DC: National Academies Press.

Marquis, J., & Huston, C. (2012). *Leadership roles and management functions in nursing.* Philadelphia, PA: Lippincott Williams & Wilkins.

Marshall, S., Harrison, J., & Flanagan, B. (2009). The teaching of a structured tool improves clarity and content of interprofessional clinical communication. *Quality and Safety in Health Care, 18*(2), 137–140.

Maxfield, D., Grenney, J., McMillan, R., Patterson, K., and Switzer, A. (2005). *Silence kills: The seven crucial conversations for healthcare.* Report from VitalSmarts, the American Association of Critical-Care Nurses, and the Association of periOperative Registered Nurses. Retrieved from http://www.silencekills.com

Maxfield, D., Grenney, J., Lavandero, R., & Groah, L. (2010). *The silent treatment: Why safety tools and checklists aren't enough to save lives.* Report from VitalSmarts, the American Association of Critical-Care Nurses, and the Association of periOperative Registered Nurses. Retrieved from http://www.silenttreatmentstudy.com

CHAPTER 15

Standard 12. Leadership

Mary-Anne D. Ponti, MS, RN, MBA, CNAA-BC, FACHE

Standard 12. Leadership. **The registered nurse demonstrates leadership in the professional practice setting and the profession.**

Definition and Explanation of the Standard

Leadership is a professional responsibility shared by all registered nurses (RNs) at all levels of practice in all settings. The Institute of Medicine (IOM, 2010) report titled *The Future of Nursing: Leading Change, Advancing Health* calls for high-quality, patient-centered health care for all, which will require a transformation of the healthcare delivery system. Nurses as leaders must be essential partners in achieving success in this initiative.

No single definition covers all of leadership's complex meanings and processes. Leadership is multifaceted and multidimensional; leadership does not "just happen" and is not limited to the few. The essence of *leadership* is the act or an instance of providing direction, guidance, and influence (Merriam-Webster, 2011; Mackenzie, 2006). It can be learned, is deliberate, and is not tied to a particular position in an organization. Many authors have defined various leadership characteristics, but no single definition is agreed on by all. The fundamental nature of leadership can be described as the ability to influence others toward accomplishing common goals. Leadership is not synonymous with management. Although their roles are often entangled, they have different functions (McCrimmon, 2010). Leaders influence people to change direction. While leadership works through influence, management works by making sound decisions, thinking, solving problems, and executing plans. Regardless of the practice setting, nurses lead and manage every day.

All RNs provide direction and guidance and exercise the process of influence every day, in every aspect of practice. Bally (2007) calls for nurses to view leadership as a collective venture. Leadership is unequivocally a professional responsibility that is shared by all RNs in all aspects of our scope of practice. RNs must accept responsibility to be leaders. According to Kotter (2007), leadership defines what the future state should look like. It establishes direction. It aligns people with a vision, motivates them, and inspires them to make it happen.

Managers focus on execution. Their skills include being catalysts, coaches, and facilitators. Leaders who are in formal management positions upgrade the function of management. Those individuals are more facilitative, nurturing, developmental, and empowering (McCrimmon, 2010). Managers who are not leaders are not able to fully engage followers, envision a future state, and exercise judgment on how to get there. The RN leads in the practice setting and profession, thereby demonstrating a blend of leadership and management.

Leadership theories have evolved over time from the Great Man and Trait Theories to more recent Transformational, Complexity, and Quantum Leadership Theories. In the classic *Leaders: Strategies for Taking Charge*, Bennis and Nanus (1997) identify four critical dimensions of empowerment that include (1) significance, (2) competence, (3) community, and (4) joy. The effective leader creates a vision that gives workers the feeling of importance. The leader supports a sense of contribution. There is an appreciation and genuine feeling of making a difference (Bennis & Nanus, 1997). Leadership in nursing exemplifying this dimension involves supporting newly licensed nurses, coaching and mentoring nurses to pursue opportunities such as clinical ladder advancement or involvement in shared governance models, and providing opportunities for others to learn through teaching or precepting. Bennis and Nanus (1997) identified four major strategies in leadership: attention through vision, meaning through communication, trust through positioning, and deployment of self.

Some say that there is a leadership crisis in America in the twenty-first century (Zinni & Koltz, 2009) and that there is a serious need for new leadership approaches to the complexity of the world and health care. Much of the emerging leadership research builds on the interactive leadership theories of the end of the twentieth century. A paradigm shift is occurring early in this century—moving from industrial-age leadership to relationship-age leadership. The leader cannot focus only on building relationships but must ensure productivity and achieve outcomes by integrating the two paradigms (Scott, 2006).

Sturm (2009) builds upon Greenleaf's (1977) servant-leadership model. Sturm concludes that servant leadership is one of the top 10 characteristics of an agile organization. It supports personal and professional growth; empowers and increases nursing leadership; and encourages collaboration, satisfaction, and retention.

Authentic leadership is another emerging leadership theory and suggests that to lead, leaders must be true to themselves and act accordingly (Stanley, 2008). This approach differs from more traditional transformational leadership that suggests a leader's vision and goals are greatly influenced by outside forces and that followers must buy in to them. Shirey (2006) describes five distinguishing characteristics of authentic leaders: purpose, values, heart, relationships, and self-discipline.

Quantum leadership is being used by leaders to better understand the dynamics of the healthcare environment. Health care and nursing are constantly changing—highly fluid, flexible, and mobile. This constant change calls for a very different and innovative approach to leadership (Porter-O'Grady & Malloch, 2007). The potential for organizational and personal conflict is high in times of rapid change, and the unexpected is becoming the norm. Therefore, leaders must be able to address and resolve conflict effectively. Using quantum leadership principles, nursing leaders work with staff members to identify common goals, build on opportunities, and empower each other to make decisions that increase organizational productivity.

The RN must consistently demonstrate specific competencies in nursing leadership, including both oversight of nursing care given by others while retaining accountability and commitment to continuous, lifelong learning. In addition, the RN must mentor colleagues, possess communication and conflict resolution skills, participate in professional organizations, and contribute to efforts that influence healthcare policy (ANA, 2010a).

Competencies for the graduate-level prepared specialty nurse and the advanced practice registered nurse include the ability to influence decision-making bodies, to provide direction to the interprofessional team, to promote advanced proactive nursing and role development, to model expert practice, and to mentor colleagues (ANA, 2010a).

Leadership in nursing is demonstrated in the professional practice setting and the profession through adhering to the professional and the legal aspects of nursing. The actions described in the scope and standards of practice serve as the underpinning of our profession, and they define our role as professional nurses. In addition, there is a legal aspect of nursing that is defined by state statute. State nurse practice acts, rules, and regulations build on our scope and standards, and they codify our obligation to society (ANA, 2010b). For example, the professional nurse demonstrates leadership in managing patient care, including the delegation to and supervision of individuals assisting in care. Consequently, the RN demonstrates leadership in nursing in the professional practice setting and the profession within a defined regulatory framework.

Application of the Standard in Practice

Education

Leadership is an essential skill that must be taught to all nursing students starting at the beginning of their curriculum, not just in a senior leadership course. Communication, conflict management, influence on health policy, prioritization, delegation, accountability, autonomy, advocacy, and so forth are all knowledge, skills, and attitudes that must be woven through the curriculum. Nurse educators have a responsibility to model leadership skills to their students in the classroom, in the clinical setting, and in professional organizations in local, state, and national arenas.

Leadership in nursing education entails vision, innovation, and an element of risk-taking in developing learning options to prepare the nurse for the needs and priorities of the future healthcare system. Education needs to continually be evaluated to ensure education changes in accordance with changes and challenges in health care. Course descriptions and objectives need to be evaluated by the RN to ensure application to practice. For example, today's nursing education environment requires a curricular framework that incorporates the core competencies of patient-centered care, team-based learning, evidence-based practice (EBP), performance improvement, and information technology (Finkelman & Kenner, 2007).

Leadership in nursing is demonstrated when RNs commit to ongoing learning, seek competency-based education, and track their professional contributions. They can accomplish their commitment by developing a professional portfolio. Uses of the portfolio include clinical-ladder advancement, role changes, job promotion or job placement, publication, and involvement in EBP and research.

Administration

As the formal leader for a nursing organization, regardless of organization or setting, the nurse administrator is the visionary, strategic planner, change agent, and practice innovator. Nurse administrators are responsible and accountable to ensure that structures and processes exist to support the RN in the professional practice setting. They influence professional practice, provide direction, promote workforce development, and ensure that nurses function within their scope of practice. They ensure that the practice is evaluated in a timely, fair, and consistent manner. Nurse administrators demonstrate leadership in nursing by ensuring that job descriptions reflect the complexity of current practice. Fundamental to the nurse administrator's ongoing professional development is promoting and supporting individual development plans. Nurses in formal leadership roles ensure that such plans are specific, timed, and measurable for the staff nurse as well as for nurses in specialty roles. Finally, nurse administrators demonstrate leadership in nursing by consciously and strategically developing future leaders. This role is exemplified through ongoing leadership development and succession planning.

Nurse administrators demonstrate leadership in nursing as they represent nursing at the highest level in an organization. They facilitate cooperative relationships with all disciplines and departments to ensure that effective quality patient care and services are consistent with professional standards, rules, and regulations of government and with regulatory agencies and corporate policies, goals, and objectives. They are accountable for continuous performance improvement as they meet or exceed nursing quality measurements and patient safety standards. Nurse administrators serve a key role in project management initiatives within the organization: they ensure that the outcomes are met for professional nursing involvement and for quality care for the healthcare consumer.

The Magnet Recognition Program® Model components of Transformational Leadership; Structural Empowerment; Exemplary Professional Practice; New Knowledge, Innovations, and Improvements; and Empirical Outcomes—all of which include the 14 Forces of Magnetism—are the foundations for nurse administrators to build programs of nursing excellence (ANCC, 2008).

Performance and Quality Improvement

Leaders in nursing oversee and ensure that quality improvement efforts are continuous, are responsive to advances in health care and changes in healthcare consumer's expectations, and are based on total commitment to the profession of nursing.

Performance improvement provides the structures and processes for measuring the quality of care and the programs to improve the quality of care provided in respective practice settings. Nurse leaders ensure that nurses participate in performance improvement. Nurses at all levels participate in and lead quality improvement by evaluating structures, processes, and outcomes of care. To improve and transform care, nurses must be committed to collecting, analyzing, and using data that can be benchmarked to excellence.

As leaders, nurses redefine and redesign care systems to meet the future needs of health care (ANCC, 2011). Nurses involved in quality improvement are specialty role nurses with specific competencies to influence decision-making bodies to improve the professional practice environment. They are pivotal in providing guidance and direction in analyzing and interpreting quality measures and outcomes. Nurses in quality and performance improvement demonstrate leadership in nursing as they assess current practices, seek EBPs, foster change, measure and report success, and ultimately improve the care of the patient.

Nurse administrators are accountable for producing empirical quality results. One of the Magnet program's core components emphasizes that organizations are in a unique position to become pioneers of the future and to demonstrate solutions to numerous problems inherent in today's health-care systems. Beyond the "what" and "how," nurse leaders must question whether those efforts have made a difference (ANCC, 2008). Improving processes in any area of care and service will improve overall outcomes in patient care; reduce unacceptable performance variation, as well as reduce patient injury and increase patient safety; and, consequently, increase a nurse's job satisfaction. Nurse leaders in this specialty need to be pioneers of the future by challenging the status quo and demonstrating solutions to problems (ANCC, 2011).

Research

The RN advances nursing autonomy and accountability by using EBP, which stresses the use of protocols and procedures substantiated by research. It involves the need for the RN to continually question practice and to seek the best available knowledge to provide care. EBP and research de-emphasize ungrounded opinion as a basis for care (The Advisory Board, 2005).

Leadership in nursing involves advancing knowledge. Enhanced knowledge, innovation, and influence on advancing practice demonstrate leadership in nursing. Professional nurses exist in many diverse roles that require a broad scope of leadership. For example, nurse educators use leadership in nursing to think, reflect, and plan how to support the evolution of competency skills needed in the clinical setting. Leadership in nursing balances the complexity of health care with the educational needs of future nurses and creates optimal learning environments. Nurses in informatics lead by designing clinical work-flow and by leading process changes in an information technology environment. Leaders in nursing ensure that the patient care needs and care delivery systems of today safely evolve into the care systems of the future. In addition, public health nurses use leadership in their role to advance the continuum of care opportunities that improve the health and well-being of individuals and communities.

Conclusion

The leadership standard states, "the registered nurse demonstrates leadership in the professional practice setting and the profession." Leadership in nursing is a responsibility of all RNs. Leadership defines what the future will look like. It aligns people and provides guidance, inspiration, and motivation. RNs are empowered to accept this responsibility through the scope and standards of practice. Leadership in nursing encompasses all areas of practice, including education, administration, quality improvement, and research, and it ensures the viability of the nursing profession.

Case Studies and Discussion Topics

Case Study 1

Stephanie is a seasoned senior staff nurse who is on an orthopedic unit and who is serving as a preceptor for a newly graduated RN named Jacob. Toward the end of the orientation, Jacob tells Stephanie that two experienced staff nurses have different patient care practices with the post-op total joint patient. Jacob informs Stephanie he does not want to get his colleagues in trouble, nor does he want them to know he has brought their differences to Stephanie's attention. He wants more than anything to fit in, but he is concerned about the differences in practice and wants to know which practice is correct.

Stephanie demonstrates the application of the leadership standard as she thanks Jacob for bringing this to her attention and acknowledges how difficult it must be for him to point out the discrepancy among the senior staff nurses. She also talks with Jacob about the importance of bringing his observations forward and about his ability to make a positive influence on patient care. Stephanie encourages and empowers Jacob to work with the unit clinical educator to search the literature on current standards of practice and to compare the literature to the current departmental policy. She coaches Jacob on how to formally assess the unit practice and to approach the issue as part of the unit performance improvement plan. She discusses the intent to address the practice variance from an educational framework.

Discussion Topics

1. What leadership competencies is Stephanie demonstrating?

2. What other actions could Stephanie take to further substantiate the application of the leadership standard?

3. What other resources could Stephanie recommend to Jacob?

Case Study 2

Mary is a nurse practitioner working in a family practice setting. The state in which she works does not allow for prescriptive authority for nurse practitioners unless they are under direct supervision of a physician. Mary demonstrates application of the leadership standard through her review of her State Nurse Practice Act. She reviews and compares this scope of practice in other states and conducts a literature review on patient outcomes with nurse practitioners who have prescriptive authority. Furthermore, Mary engages with other nurse practitioners and her state representative to submit legislation to allow independent prescriptive authority. Finally, Mary testifies on her support of the bill. In her testimony, Mary speaks to the need to support nurses in their ability to function to their fullest level of education and licensure.

Discussion Topics

1. What barriers do you anticipate Mary will experience with her initiative?

2. What leadership competencies is Mary demonstrating?

3. How could Mary further influence the professional practice environment?

References and Other Sources

The Advisory Board Company. (2005). *Evidenced-based nursing practice: Instilling rigor into clinical practice.* Washington, DC: Author.

American Nurses Association (ANA). (2010a). *Nursing: Scope and standards of practice* (2nd ed.). Silver Spring, MD: Nursesbooks.org.

American Nurses Association (ANA). (2010b). *Nursing's social policy statement: The essence of the profession.* Silver Spring, MD: Nursesbooks.org.

American Nurses Credentialing Center (ANCC). (2008). *A new model for ANCC's Magnet Recognition Program®.* Silver Spring, MD: Author.

American Nurses Credentialing Center (ANCC). (2011). Magnet overview: Announcing a new model for ANCC's Magnet Recognition Program®. Retrieved from http://www.nursecredentialing.org/MagnetModel.aspx

Bally, J. M. G. (2007). The role of nursing leadership in creating a mentoring culture in acute care environments. *Nursing Economics, 25*(3), 143–148.

Bennis, W., & Nanus, B. (1997). *Leaders: Strategies for taking charge.* New York, NY: Harper Collins Publishers.

Finkelman, A., & Kenner, C. (2007). *Teaching IOM: Implications of the Institute of Medicine reports for nursing education* (2nd ed.). Silver Spring, MD: Nursesbooks.org.

Greenleaf, R. K. (1977). *Servant leadership: A journey in the nature of legitimate power and greatness.* New York, NY: Paulist.

Institute of Medicine (IOM). (2010). *The future of nursing: Leading change, advancing health.* Retrieved from www.iom.edu/nursing.

Kotter, J. P. (2007). Leading change: Why change fails. *Harvard Business Review, 85*(1), 96–103.

Mackenzie, K. (2006). The LAMPE theory of organizational leadership. In F. Yammarino and F. Dansereau (Eds.), *Research in multi-level issues* (Vol. 5). Oxford, UK: Elsevier Science.

McCrimmon, M. (2010). Reinventing leadership and management. *Ivey Business Journal, May/June 2010.* Retrieved from http://www.iveybusinessjournal.com/topics/leadership/reinventing-leadership-and-management

Merriam-Webster. (2012). Online dictionary. Springfield, MA: Merriam-Webster. Retrieved from http://www.merriam-webster.com/dictionary/leading?show=0&t=1304279227

Porter-O'Grady, T., & Malloch, K. (2007). *Quantum leadership: A resource for health care innovation* (2nd ed.). Sudbury, MA: Jones & Bartlett.

Scott, K. T. (2006). The gifts of leadership. In B. Marquis & C. Huston (Eds.), *Leadership roles and management functions in nursing* (2009, p. 60). Philadelphia, PA: Lippincott Williams & Wilkins.

Shirey, M. R. (2006). Authentic leadership: Foundation of a health work environment. *American Journal of Critical Care, 20*(3), 130–133. Retrieved from http://www.ncbi.nlm.nih.gov/pubmed/16632768

Stanley, D. (2008). Congruent leadership: Values in action. *Journal of Nursing Management, 16*(5), 519–524.

Sturm, B. A. (2009). Principles of servant-leadership in community health nursing: Management issues and behaviors discovered in ethnographic research. *Home Health Care Management and Practice, 21*(2), 82–89.

Zinni, T., & Koltz, T. (2009). *Leading the charge: Leadership lessons from the battlefield to the boardroom.* New York, NY: Palgrave Macmillan.

CHAPTER 16

Standard 13. Collaboration

Pamela Brown, PhD, RN

Standard 13. Collaboration. **The registered nurse collaborates with the healthcare consumers, family, and others in the conduct of nursing practice.**

Definition and Explanation of the Standard

The word *collaborate* comes from Latin origins, *com* (together) and *laborare* (to labor), to exert together, to work one with another, to cooperate, especially in a joint effort toward mutual goals (Merriam-Webster, 2011). In nursing and medicine, Baggs and Schmitt (1998) defined collaboration more narrowly as "nurses and physicians cooperatively working together, sharing responsibility for solving problems, and making decisions to formulate and carry out plans for patient care" (p. 74). Over time, the definition has broadened to include multiple professions and a variety of stakeholders.

Collaboration, as a concept, is not new to nursing or health care and continues to be an essential element in safe and high-quality patient-care outcomes (IOM, 2010). Although collaboration is a common and an essential part of everyday practice, much variation in outcomes continues to exist in health care (Sullivan, 1998; IOM, 2010). The ongoing challenge to achieve positive outcomes through collaboration rests with the "co" part of collaboration, in working together effectively toward a mutual goal. This approach takes "intentional knowledge sharing and joint responsibility" (Lindeke & Sieckert, 2005, p. 1).

Collaboration is multifaceted and complex. It occurs in rapid one-on-one encounters and in long-term projects, as well as electronically with no face-to-face interactions. It occurs within short- and long-term relationships. In nursing, it includes descriptors, such as *intra*professional (nurse to nurse or within the profession) and *inter*professional (nurse to other professionals or between the professions). It also includes nurse to healthcare consumers and external agencies.

The Interprofessional Education Collaborative Expert Panel (2011)—representing the American Association of Colleges of Nursing, the American Association of College of Osteopathic Medicine, the American Association of Colleges of Pharmacy, the American Dental Education Association, the Association of Medical Colleges, and the Association of Schools of Public Health—released a report addressing core competencies for interprofessional collaborative practice. The panel proposed four domains of care competencies needed to provide integrated, high-quality patient care, and it identified 38 specific, individual-level, core, interprofessional competencies that are across the domains and are necessary for future health professionals. They recommend that health professionals do the following:

- Assert values and ethics of interprofessional practice by placing the interests, dignity, and respect of patients at the center of healthcare delivery and by embracing the cultural diversity and differences of healthcare teams.

- Leverage the unique roles and responsibilities of interprofessional partners to appropriately assess and address the healthcare needs of patients and populations served.

- Communicate with patients, families, communities, and other health professionals in support of a team approach to preventing disease and disability, maintaining health, and treating disease.

- Perform effectively in various team roles to deliver patient- and population-centered care that is safe, timely, efficient, effective, and equitable.

Registered nurses (RNs) are expected to have competencies (ANA, 2010) that encompass using interpersonal communication and teambuilding skills to partner with others to effect change and manage conflict. Nurses must participate in documenting an integrated plan of care that focuses on outcomes and decisions related to care and delivery of services and that indicates mutual communication with healthcare consumers. An RN also engages in collaborative reasoning and decision-making. Collaborative reasoning refers to the "nurturing of a consensual approach toward the interpretation of examination finding, the setting of goals and priorities, and the implementation and progression of treatment" (Edwards, Jones, Higgs, Trede, & Jensen, 2004, p. 72).

Collaborative reasoning requires RNs to have ample depth of knowledge in their own discipline and clear understanding of the patient, family, community, and population, along with adequate knowledge about other disciplines' scope of practice. Collaborative decision-making ethically supports (1) the right of persons and communities to participate in making decisions affecting their health and (2) the importance of ensuring informed consent. Collaborative decision-making emphasizes the partnership among nurses; other professionals; and patients, families, communities, and populations with the mutual goal of improving patient safety and outcomes.

In summary, an RN is expected to be proficient in collaborating with healthcare professionals and to be an effective part of an interprofessional healthcare team that provides high-quality and safe patient care to individuals and populations.

Competencies expected of the graduate-level prepared specialty nurse and the advanced practice registered nurse (APRN) encompass establishing, improving, and sustaining collaborative relationships, as well as partnering with other disciplines (ANA, 2010). Graduate nurses are key leaders in collaborative discussions that improve healthcare consumer outcomes. An APRN is expected to be proficient in collaboration among healthcare professionals and to effectively implement high-quality and safe patient care at the systems level and at the level of the individual, family, community, or population. All nurses must become proficient in working in collaborative and interdependent relationships and in fostering an interprofessional team approach to patient care.

Common interprofessional collaborations for both levels of nursing practice include population-based disease management, such as diabetes, congestive heart failure, and pneumonia. Multiple professionals are involved in managing the care of such patient populations, including physicians, nurses in home care and acute-care settings, nurse case managers, social workers, pharmacists, respiratory therapists, and physical therapists. All of those professionals, plus the patient and family, are crucial contributors to safe and quality care outcomes.

The nurse's knowledge, skills, and attitude determine how effective he or she is at collaboration. Nurses need knowledge to assess their collaboration expertise and to understand the scope and roles of other professionals, and they need strong communication skills to promote collaboration that is within interprofessional teams and that improves safety and quality of consumer healthcare (QSEN, 2011). The skills necessary include commitment to lifelong learning and self-development.

Competency in one's own practice, whether as a team member or leader, is essential in integrating professional contributions to consumer health goals. To lead or participate in designing systems that support collaborative practice, nurses must act with integrity and respect toward other's differing viewpoints. They must communicate in styles that minimize risks associated with handoffs among providers and across transitions in care. And nurses must diminish risks associated with authority gradients among health professionals.

Finally, nurses need to be able to welcome differences that may lead to disagreements and conflicts and, at the same time, appreciate that safe quality patient care is the imperative among all providers and caregivers. Nurses must respect that the healthcare consumer is central to the collaborative process, because nurses value the influence of system solutions to achieve effective collaborative practices (QSEN, 2010). Baggs (2005) identifies networking as the most crucial behavior associated with collaboration. Leaders need to inspire stakeholders, and they need a vision to reach shared purpose and mutual goals.

Application of the Standard in Practice

Education

To align with the IOM recommendations, nursing education must include interprofessional team learning experiences. Interprofessional team learning offers students practice in teamwork and collaborative reasoning and decision-making. Benner, Sutphen, Leonard, and Day (2010) found "almost no interdisciplinary learning or practice opportunities for students," and believe "practice in an interdisciplinary setting can help students work more effectively on a healthcare team as well as better integrate knowledge, skilled know-how, and ethical comportment in practice" (p. 229). Interprofessional classroom, clinical, laboratory, and simulation experiences are all effective ways to foster collaboration and appreciation for contributions of all professionals to the team. In 2011, national experts convened to develop strategies that healthcare educators could use to implement the IPEC (Interprofessional Education Collaborative) core competencies and move the healthcare educational system toward collaborative health professionals. Those strategies include the following:

1. Communicate and disseminate the core competencies to key stakeholders—academic deans, policy makers, and healthcare leaders—and launch an education campaign that makes the critical link between using collaborative healthcare teams and providing high-quality, safe, and cost-sensitive treatment.

2. Prepare faculty members for teaching students how to work effectively as part of a team, and encourage all health professions to use the competencies in their fields.

3. Develop metrics for interprofessional education and collaborative care to help advance team-based competencies in teaching and practice.

4. Forge partnerships among the academic community, healthcare providers, and government agencies to advance interprofessional education. (AACN, 2011)

Combining teamwork and collaboration, the Quality and Safety Education for Nurses (QSEN) program reaffirms that nurses must "function effectively within nursing and interprofessional teams, fostering open communication, mutual respect, and shared decision-making to achieve quality patient care" (QSEN, 2011). Collaboration between nursing education and nursing practice to assess gaps between education and practice creates individualized orientation and residency programs for new graduates. Those programs both assist the transition of new graduates to "competent" practitioners and reduce nurse turnover in practice settings.

Administration

As healthcare delivery systems experience escalating demands, increasing complexity, and diminishing resources, nursing administrators must create environments that promote interprofessional collaborative practice. That practice focuses on interprofessional communication and interprofessional evidence-based care and includes all stakeholders and multiple professionals in the development and organization of patient care.

Key examples of interprofessional communication are transitions in care and nurse–physician collaboration. Transitions are essential processes that protect patient safety and improve the coordination of care. If transitions are handled poorly, patient errors (harm) increase. Transition reports are a collaborative process involving the relinquishing of responsibility for a patient or group of patients by one person or group, the acceptance of responsibility for that patient or group of patients, and the sharing of information about the patient or group of patients (Wilson, Randell, Galliers, & Woodward, 2009).

Communication or sharing of information between physicians and nurses is a critical element in the collaborative process and is key to safe, high-quality patient care. In 2004, The Joint Commission disseminated a sentinel event illustrating that communication issues among care providers were identified as the root cause of infant death and injury in 72% of 47 cases reviewed. In 2008, another sentinel event was distributed; it pointed out that poor interprofessional communication is a major contributor to medical errors and resultant harm to patients (Colombo, 2009). Nursing administrators must develop systems, policies and processes, education, and accountabilities for interprofessional collaborative communication in these and other situations.

Interprofessional team-based, evidence-based practice has been shown to provide improved efficiency and quality of service, decreased cost with improved patient outcomes, and increased job satisfaction. The review by Medves et al. (2010, p. 80) asserts that "collaborative team practice and the implementation of practice guidelines are promising approaches in healthcare delivery." Currently, there are multiple approaches to developing and implementing evidence-based care guidelines, many remain in silos (uniprofessional) or are discipline specific. The development of or adoption of team-based, evidence-based guidelines provides interprofessional teams with a more unified approach to care. According to Medves, et al. (2010, p. 79), team-based health care and practice are "widely argued to provide not only improved efficiency and quality of service, but also cost reductions and increased job satisfaction." Nurse administrators must lead improvement initiatives and must build interprofessional teams focused on providing team-based, evidence-based care that improves healthcare consumer safety and quality of care.

When revising or creating patient care delivery services, nurse administrators involve all relevant stakeholders, such as multiple disciplines and department representatives, front-line staff members, patients, families, and architects. The administrator must create a safe environment with mutual respect and must address the power differences among the members. Equality between professionals and other team members is one of the basic character-istics of positive collaborative team-based practice, and this process is greatly impeded when power differences are not addressed (Martin-Rodriquez, Beaulieu, D'Amour, & Ferrada-Videla, 2005).

One way to address the power differences is to build consensus about "how" the team will interact. The group agrees on "rules" of engagement, such as "leave your title at the door," "every individual is a valued member of the team," "each person provides valuable information and will be given an opportunity to talk without interruption," "every opinion is honored," or "cell phones set to off or vibrate," and so forth. Once rules are agreed upon, the leader keeps them in the forefront of the participants and refers to them as needed. Mutual goals are usually established early and may be used as a reference to return the group to its mutual purpose.

Performance and Quality Improvement

Virtually all nurses are involved as front-line care providers in some manner in quality improvement practices. Although one nurse does make a difference in improving quality and safe patient care, an interprofessional team–based, evidence-based approach to improving and sustaining high-quality and safe patient care must happen at the system level. For example, an interprofessional team is essential in reducing the number of medication errors because such errors are outside the scope of any one profession. Leaders and staff members from nursing, pharmacy, supply chain, financial services, and other healthcare professionals are needed to effectively analyze the problems or barriers and to enact quality improvement team–based, evidence-based strategies that include system changes (Hall, Barnsteiner, & Moore, 2008).

Although newer nurses are introduced to quality improvement theory and tools, the current nursing workforce is made up of four generations, and many nurses have no background in quality improvement theory or tools. All nurses need to acquire knowledge, skills, and attitudes that lead to competency in the areas identified by QSEN: patient-centered care; col-laboration; team-based, evidence-based practice; quality improvement and safety; and informatics.

Research

Historically, requirements for terminal degrees in nursing focused on conduct-ing individual research and developing an individual program of research. In more recent years, both team-based research and research programs have gained acceptance. Today, interprofessional research teams that are focused on team-based, evidence-based best practices represent the preferred approach to close the "quality chasm" identified by the IOM (2001). To advance improvement science in nursing and health care, collaborations for team-based, evidence-based research studies are needed.

The interprofessional research team of Naylor et al. (2007, p. 72) reported that their current study involving care coordination for cognitively impaired older adults and their caregivers had been "substantially informed by our team's program of research over the past 18 years." This research by Naylor and her team (2007, 2009) concentrates on closing the quality chasm in the transitional care for older adults by conducting team-based, evidence-based research and by translating research into practice. Other large, evidence-based, interprofessional team interventions have been developed to deal with transition issues for the care of the elderly population, such as the Care Transitions Program® (2011). These critical, team-based interventions are based on meeting two key priorities: communicating and transferring critical elements of the patient's care plan and executing essential steps before and after transferring a patient.

Another large collaborative effort is by the Improvement Science Research Network (ISRN). The ISRN's purpose (ISRN, 2011) is "to advance the scientific foundation for quality improvement, safety and efficiency through transdisciplinary research addressing healthcare systems, patient-centeredness, and integration of evidence into practice." To accomplish this goal, a steering council, composed of 16 expert members from multiple disciplines, has been developed. The coordinating center is housed at the University of Texas Health Science Center–San Antonio. This center allows interprofessional research teams to conduct research in multiple and diverse clinical settings and to communicate through the Internet. The ISRN has also partnered with the Institute of Integration of Medicine and Science to further reduce barriers to research and to strengthen the science of quality improvement. The ISRN research priorities are as follows:

1. Coordination and transitions of care.

2. High performing clinical systems and microsystems approaches to improvement.

3. Evidence-based quality improvement and best practice.

4. Learning organizations and culture of quality and safety.

The Essential Guide to Nursing Practice

Conclusion

No man is an island, entire of itself; every man is a piece of the continent,
a piece of the main. . . .

—John Donne

Meditation XVII, 1572–1631

The poet John Donne wrote eloquently about each individual being part of the whole. Each standard is also part of the whole. Nurses need to realize that no standard stands alone. To be proficient in collaboration, one must also be proficient in communication and teamwork. Effective interpersonal communication is integral to teamwork and collaboration. Each nurse has the moral and ethical responsibility to continue to hone his or her skills in interpersonal communication, teamwork, and collaboration, just as one diligently updates and upgrades one's theoretical knowledge.

Case Studies and Discussion Topics

Case Study 1

Judd is a novice nurse working on an orthopedic surgical unit and experiencing change-of-shift patient rounds as a way of transitioning patient care on his unit. He takes notes, but rounds progress very quickly. He routinely finds that he is later missing important information and often loses efficiency by seeking or clarifying information from nurses on the previous shift and by contacting other disciplines for information not shared during change-of-shift patient rounds. He seeks advice from other nurses on the unit and finds that he is not alone in his concerns. Judd discusses his concerns with his immediate supervisor and is encouraged to put together a task force to improve the hand-off process, thereby increasing patient safety and continuity of care.

Judd demonstrates competency in collaboration by gathering nurses from different shifts and including respiratory and physical therapy representatives and a nutritionist on the initial task force. Judd's supervisor supports his initiative and coaches him in building consensus among group members. Judd demonstrates competency in collaboration by helping the group members state their common purpose and set mutual goals. He seeks group consensus on how all voices will be heard and valued, including clarifying scope and roles of each discipline. Once the group has an initial to-do list, Judd reviews shared responsibilities in reporting back to the group. The outcome is that this task force recommends that the unit adopt a hand-off checklist and include key disciplines in change-of-shift rounds.

Discussion Topics

1. How could Judd have included patient and families in his task force?

2. Can you state the common purpose for this task force?

3. Can you write two common goals for this task force?

4. What system-level processes might be involved in implementing the recommendations?

Case Study 2

Deloris is a master's prepared clinical nurse who is leading an evidence-based practice team that manages the care of Stanley, an elderly male who is not expected to live through the night. His family requests last rites for him. The bedside nurse notifies the priest on call, and he is unavailable. She then notifies the supervisor (a nun) and is told that the nun is busy in the pharmacy. The family asks the bedside nurse to pray a common Roman Catholic prayer for them, but she is unfamiliar with the desired prayer. She stays with the patient and his family; unfortunately, no one prays the desired prayer nor conducts last rites for Stanley before his death. As the team reflects on this event, they conclude that a pamphlet of diverse yet common prayers would be beneficial for healthcare providers. They want to couple this with an education module to facilitate use of this resource.

Discussion Topics

1. What members (disciplines and stakeholders) need to be recruited for this project?

2. What common purpose should Deloris propose?

3. Can you write three mutual goals?

4. What knowledge, skills, and attitudes does Deloris's team need to demonstrate during this collaborative effort?

5. How would Deloris demonstrate that this project is evidence based and centered on the patient?

6. What are some systems and processes that Deloris's team might need to address for this project?

References and Other Sources

American Association of Colleges of Nursing (AACN). (2011). AACN, health educators, foundations release competencies and action strategies for interprofessional education. Retrieved from http://www.aacn.nche.edu/news/articles/2011/ipec

American Nurses Association (ANA). (2010). *Nursing: Scope and standards of practice* (2nd ed.). Silver Spring, MD: Nursesbooks.org.

Baggs, J. G. (2005). Overview and summary: Partnerships and collaboration: What skills are needed? *Online Journal of Issues in Nursing, 10913734, 10*(1).

Baggs, J. G., & Schmitt, M. H. (1998). Collaboration between nurses and physicians. *Image: Journal of Nursing Scholarship, 20,* 145–149.

Bainbridge, L., Nasmith, L., Orchard, C., & Wood, V. (2010). Competencies for interprofessional collaboration. *Journal of Physical Therapy Education, 24*(1), 6–11.

Benner, P., Sutphen, M., Leonard, V., & Day, L. (2010). *Educating nurses: A call for radical change.* San Francisco, CA: Jossey-Bass.

The Care Transitions Program®. (2011). An interdisciplinary team approach to improving transitions across sites of geriatric care. Retrieved from http://www.caretransitions.org

Clark, E., Burkett, K., & Stanko-Lopp, D. (2009). Let evidence guide every new decision (LEGEND): An evidence evaluation system for point of care clinicians and guideline development teams. *Journal of Evaluation in Clinical Practice, 15,* 1054–1060.

Coleman, E. A. (2003). Falling through the cracks: Challenges and opportunities for improving transitional care for persons with continuous complex care needs. *Journal of American Geriatric Society, 51,* 549–555.

Coleman, E. A., Smith, J. D., Frank, J. C., Joon-Min, S., Parry, C., & Kramer, A. M. (2004). Preparing patients and caregivers to participate in care delivered across settings: The care transitions intervention. *Journal of American Geriatric Society, 52,* 1817–1825.

Colombo, C. (2009). Nurse–physician summit: Fostering communication, collaboration, and commitment. *Nursing for Women's Health, 13*(6), 511–514.

Dedhia, P., Kravey, S., Bulger, J., Hinson, T., Sridharan, A., Kolodner, K., Wright, S., & Howell, E. (2009). A quality improvement intervention to facilitate the transition of older adults from three hospitals back to their homes. *Journal of the American Geriatrics Society, 57,* 1540–1546.

Edwards, I., Jones, M., Higgs, J., Trede, F., & Jensen, G. (2004). What is collaborative reasoning? *Advances in Physiotherapy, 6,* 70–83.

Hall, L. W., Barnsteiner, J. H., & Moore, S. M. (2008). Quality and nursing: Moving from a concept to a core competency. *Urologic Nursing, 28*(6), 417–425.

Improvement Science Research Network. (2011). Retrieved from http://www.improvementscienceresearch.net

Institute of Medicine (IOM). (2010). *The future of nursing: Leading change, advancing health.* Washington, DC: National Academies Press.

Institute of Medicine (IOM). (2005). *Quality through collaboration: The future of rural health.* Washington, DC: National Academies Press.

Institute of Medicine (IOM). (2001). Crossing the quality chasm: A new health system for the 21st century. Washington, DC: National Academies Press.

Interprofessional Education Collaborative Expert Panel. (2011). *Report of an expert panel.* Washington, DC: Interprofessional Education Collaborative.

Lindeke, L., & Sieckert, A. M. (2005). Nurse–physician workplace collaboration. *Online Journal of Issues in Nursing, 10*(1).

Martin-Rodriguez, L. S., Beaulieu, M. D., D'Amour, D., & Ferrada-Videla, M. (2005). The determinants of successful collaboration: A review of theoretical and empirical studies. *Journal of Interprofessional Care, 19*(2), 132–147.

Medves, J., Godfrey, C., Turner, C., Paterson, M., Harrison, M., MacKenze, L., & Durnado, P. (2010). Systematic review of practice guideline dissemination and implementation strategies for healthcare teams and team based practice. *International Journal of Evidence-Based Healthcare, 8,* 79–89.

Merriam-Webster's Online Dictionary (11th ed.). (2011). Springfield, MA: Merriam-Webster. Retrieved from http://www.merriam-webster.com/dictionary/collaborate

Naylor, M. D., Feldman, P. H., Keating, S., Koren, M. J., Kurtzman, E. T., Maccoy, M. C., & Krakauer, R. (2009). Translating research into practice: Transitional care for older adults. *Journal of Evaluation in Clinical Practice, 15,* 1164–1170.

Naylor, M. D., Hirschman, K. B., Bowles, K. H., Bixby, M. B., Konick-McMahon, J., & Stephens, C. (2007). Care coordination for cognitively impaired older adults and their caregivers. *Home Health Care Services Quarterly, 26,* 57–78. Available online at http://hhc.haworthpress.com

Nolan, T. W. (2007). Execution of strategic improvement initiatives to produce system-level results. IHI Innovation Series white paper. Cambridge, MA: Institute for Healthcare Improvement. Available online at http://www.IHI.org

Quality and Safety Education for Nurses (QSEN). (2011). Retrieved from http://www.qsen.org

Sullivan, T. J. (1998). *Collaboration: A health care imperative.* New York, NY: McGraw Hill Companies.

Wilson, S., Randell, R., Galliers, J., & Woodward, P. (2009). *Reconceptualizing clinical handover: Information sharing for situation awareness.* Otaniemi, Finland: European Conference on Cognitive Ergonomics.

CHAPTER 17

Standard 14. Professional Practice Evaluation

Joanne V. Hickey, PhD, RN, ACNP-BC, FAAN

Standard 14. Professional Practice Evaluation. **The registered nurse evaluates her or his own nursing practice in relation to professional practice standards and guidelines, relevant statutes, rules, and regulations.**

Definition and Explanation of the Standard

Evaluation is the process of determining the progress toward attainment of expected outcomes, including effectiveness of care (ANA, 2010). The professional registered nurse (RN) has a responsibility to engage in evaluation activities to maintain and enhance her or his professional performance as part of accountability to the healthcare consumer and to the profession. As part of the evaluation process, the RN identifies and monitors official, valid, and reliable authoritative sources of information for professional practice standards, guidelines, statutes, rules, and regulations that serve as a basis for evaluation of professional performance. Moreover, the RN assumes responsibility and accountability for meeting the criteria for ethical, legal, and professional standards of practice.

While engaging in periodic and systematic self-evaluation of professional performance, the RN compares personal knowledge, skills, and abilities to established criteria. Such an evaluation begins with the collection of many forms of evidence through formal and informal sources (e.g., reflection, performance evaluations, oral situational feedback, and other sources) with the goal of fostering professional growth and development. The RN seeks input related to professional performance from multiple external sources, such as colleagues, supervisors, mentors, patients, families, and other stakeholders. The RN also uses the information from evaluations to create an action plan for professional growth and development in accordance with professional standards. In fact, the RN participates in multiple activities to evaluate performance in relation to established criteria (e.g., competency assessment and continuing education assessment of knowledge).

By seeking educational opportunities to develop and enhance competencies, the RN engages in professional activities to maintain accurate and current knowledge of requirements for professional practice. In addition, the RN recognizes a collegial responsibility to assist peers in maintaining and developing their professional competencies. To fulfill this responsibility, the RN provides informal constructive feedback (e.g., situational feedback, overall performance feedback, and suggestions for growth and development) to peers.

There are some differences when applying the standard professional practice evaluation to the graduate-level prepared nurse or advanced practice registered nurse (APRN). Those nurses are held to a higher standard of implementation of professional practice evaluation, a standard that reflects their education, roles, responsibilities, and accountability. While drawing on specialty advanced practice performance criteria and other standards for graduate-level prepared nurses, the RN with graduate-level education seeks feedback about her or his professional practice from a broader range of constituents than does the generalist, such as nursing peers, professional colleagues, collaborators, mentors, healthcare consumers, and others. The evaluation includes the effect of her or his professional practice on local, regional, national, and international levels, as well as the effect of contributions to the profession of nursing. She or he is able to translate collected feedback into a career development plan that is periodically reviewed and updated. The APRN or graduate-level prepared nurse seeks opportunities for professional growth and development on the regional, national, and international level. She or he assumes responsibility for lifelong learning as a commitment to providing the highest quality of care to individual patients and populations and to contributing to the nursing profession.

Application of the Standard in Practice

Education

Professional practice evaluation content should be included in planning and developing the nursing curriculum, the didactic and clinical evaluation tools, and the professional portfolio. Content on scope and standards of professional nursing practice, nursing's code of ethics legal requirements for practice, regulation of professional nursing practice, and career planning and development should be included as threads throughout the curriculum in both didactic and clinical practice experiences. Students should be provided opportunities for inclusion of this content to enhance clinical reasoning competencies in professional practice evaluation. As members (for parallelism) of the nursing profession, students must understand and embrace a personal responsibility and accountability for lifelong learning and for updating their knowledge throughout their careers.

An important component of learning about evaluation is understanding both peer- and self-evaluation. *Peer evaluation* includes both evaluating and being evaluated by peers. Both processes are conducted respectfully with the goal of providing another perspective gained from professional relationships and knowledge about the performance of the person being evaluated. *Self-evaluation* requires one to know what to evaluate, how to collect that data, how to analyze and evaluate the data, and what to do with the findings. It requires a level of objectivity and self-knowledge about performance as compared to expected competencies and standards. Through learning about the development and maintenance of a professional portfolio, students are given the tools to document learning and to map their professional careers.

Administration

The standards of practice and culture of an organization for job descriptions, performance appraisals, individual professional development, and support create the framework for the nurse to engage in professional practice evaluation as a planned growth experience. Organizational administration should use evidence-based and best practices in the evaluation processes. The organization that employs professional RNs has a responsibility to include standards of professional practice in its annual performance appraisals. The organization also assumes responsibility for providing supervisory personnel who are competent in evaluating, coaching, and mentoring professional RNs who, in turn, can identify areas for growth and can provide support for professional development. A comprehensive evaluation of professional RNs includes periodic competency evaluation of critical knowledge, skills, and abilities to support competent care for patients (Twedell, 2011).

Individualized development plans (IDPs) have been used in business and industry and are now being implemented in health care. An IDP is an individually tailored plan that describes objectives and activities for the nurse's career development and that is designed to enhance a nurse's knowledge, skills, and competencies. It can be used in a number of ways. The most common way is for the nurse and employer (e.g., direct supervisor) to identify specific areas most important to both of them. This information serves as a basis for developing an action plan to achieve the goals. The IDP serves as a map for professional growth that can be reviewed periodically to determine progress.

Performance and Quality Improvement

To support quality and high-level performance, an organization should include periodic assessment of critical knowledge, skills, and abilities for competent nursing practice and care. To assist professional RNs, peer review mechanisms should be available to address deviations from established criteria for professional practice. In addition, counseling services must be available to assist the professional RN in correcting deviations from standards of care and performance. Nurses must recognize their advocacy role to speak up when they observe deviations from accepted standards of practice or care (ANA, 2001). They must also know how to give feedback to others in constructive ways that are designed to improve performance and patient safety. Those types of communication skills should be taught and practiced (e.g., through role-playing) so that the nurse is comfortable with addressing such situations when they occur.

Research

So the evidence base for professional practice evaluation can develop and grow, the profession must support research on professional practice evaluation of professional RNs from all levels of education and professional responsibility (Polit & Beck, 2008). Currently, the state of the science about key competencies and about how to evaluate competency is very limited. Along with national imperatives for quality and safety, the profession needs to stimulate and support research on professional performance and its evaluation. Research can be stimulated and supported in the work environment through journal clubs, periodic research days, and bulletin boards highlighting important studies. In addition, partnerships with academia to assist with research initiatives are well-proven methods to stimulate research.

RNs should be expected to participate to the level of their education and experience with clinical research. Empowering nurses must be encouraged so they can raise clinical questions related to their practice; such questions can become the basis for studies that can improve the processes and outcomes of care and practice. Creating a culture of clinical inquiry both supports research and stimulates analysis and evaluation of current practices and care. Including the expectation of participation in research in a nurse's annual performance evaluation underscores that the profession and organization value research and expect professional nurses to participate in building the knowledge base of the profession.

Conclusion

The expectation for the RN to evaluate her or his nursing practice in relation to multiple professional practice standards, guidelines, relevant statutes, rules, and regulation is the framework for demonstrating responsibility and accountability for providing competent, high-quality care for patients and for contributing to the profession of nursing. Commitment to professional practice evaluation as a basis for professional growth and development is an integrated activity shared by education, administration, quality improvement, and research components of the profession. However, the RN assumes the ultimate responsibility to participate in evaluation activities that will achieve and maintain the highest level of professional performance.

Case Studies and Discussion Topics

Case Study 1
During the orientation of a group of newly hired RNs at a healthcare facility, the speaker tells the group members that they have a professional responsibility to evaluate their own professional performance. An RN in the audience raises her hand and asks how she should go about evaluating her professional performance.

Discussion Topics
1. What general advice would you give her about evaluation?

2. What specific advice would you give her regarding collection of data?

3. Once she collected the data, what would you advise her to do with the data to help her in planning for competency and professional development?

4. Who could help her with her professional development?

Case Study 2

You are the charge nurse on a unit. An RN on your unit has confided in you that she is concerned about the omission in care that she has observed in an RN who has recently transferred to your unit. She is concerned that the omissions in care are jeopardizing the safety of patients.

Discussion Topics

1. In exploring this situation with the RN, how would you respond?

2. What questions would you ask?

3. What advice would you give her?

4. Now that you have been made aware of these concerns related to patients, what is your responsibility?

References

American Nurses Association (ANA). (2001). *Code of Ethics for Nurses with interpretive statements*. Washington, DC: Author.

American Nurses Association (ANA). (2010). *Nursing: Scope and standards of practice* (2nd ed.). Silver Spring, MD: Author.

Polit, D. E., & Beck, C. T. (2008). *Nursing research: Generating and assessing evidence for nursing practice* (8th ed.) (pp. 1–27). Philadelphia, PA: Wolters Kluwer Health, Lippincott William & Wilkins.

Twedell, D. M. (2011). Selecting, developing, and evaluating staff. In P. S. Yoder-Wise (Ed.), *Leading and managing in nursing* (5th ed.) (pp. 293–306). St. Louis, MO: Elsevier Mosby.

The Essential Guide to Nursing Practice

CHAPTER 18

Standard 15. Resource Utilization

Kathleen M. White, PhD, RN, NEA-BC, FAAN

Standard 15. Resource Utilization. **The registered nurse utilizes appropriate resources to plan and provide nursing services that are safe, effective, and financially responsible.**

Definition and Explanation of the Standard

Resource utilization is the amount of a good or service consumed or the pattern of use of a good or service within a specified time. The basic resources needed to provide a good or service are financial, human, technological, and physical.

Appropriate resource utilization in health care is everyone's responsibility. A nurse, as a major healthcare provider, is increasingly held accountable for resource use and the costs of patient care. Nurses have a key role in determining healthcare resource needs, obtaining those resources, and often participating in the allocation of scarce resources. Quality care remains the goal in health care, and outcomes-focused plans of care have been shown to contain resource utilization and to enhance quality. Resource utilization is a dynamic process; nurses and other healthcare providers must be able to identify the costs of care or the costs of an illness in order to identify necessary resources and to manage resource utilization in health care (Dunham-Taylor & Pinczek, 2006).

Over the years, the healthcare system has been challenged with resource utilization and with, as the standard states, "providing services that are safe, effective, and financially responsible." The development of Medicare's prospective payment system or diagnosis-related groups in 1983 was the first attempt to contain costs and to address healthcare resource utilization by specifically targeting length of stay. Nurses should consider several recent models of healthcare delivery that have focused on resource utilization by trying to achieve an appropriate balance of cost, resources, and quality.

Managed care focused on resource utilization, coordination of appropriate care, attention to preventive health care, and conservation of resources through the management of care by a healthcare provider or insurer. Case management, another technique that focuses on resource utilization, is a collaborative process that assesses, plans, implements, coordinates, monitors, and evaluates the options and services required to meet the client's health and human services needs. It is characterized by advocacy, communication, and resource management, and it promotes quality and cost-effective interventions and outcomes (Commission for Case Manager Certification, 2011).

The stated goal of case management is to coordinate patient care resources. The Institute of Medicine (IOM, 2001) report titled *Crossing the Quality Chasm: A New Health Report for the 21st Century* described the U.S. healthcare system as "poorly organized to meet the challenges at hand." In addition, it discusses the system's cumbersome processes and waste of resources that lead to safety concerns, lack of appropriate care, and loss of information. The report recommended six aims for improvement—all with a critical resource utilization foundation—that are built around the need for health care to be safe, timely, effective, efficient, equitable, and patient-centered.

The latest and evolving innovation in healthcare resource utilization is the accountable care organization (ACO). The ACO, a group of providers of services and suppliers who work together to manage and coordinate care, will be responsible for the patient's entire episode of illness across the continuum. Nurses will have a major role in the evolution of those ACOs. Their expertise in resource identification and care coordination will be valuable to the success of the ACO (Center for Medicare and Medicaid Services, 2012; Gold, 2011).

All nurses must participate in resource utilization in health care. This critical knowledge is important in everyday nursing practice for clinical decision-making. As patient advocates, the registered nurse (RN) has an important role in assessing the healthcare consumer's and family's needs, identifying desired outcomes, and assisting them to negotiate and navigate resources for their health care across the continuum. This role includes evaluating the evidence and determining and securing the appropriate level of care and services necessary to meet the consumer's desired outcomes. The nurse advocates for

The Essential Guide to Nursing Practice

appropriate evaluation and use of therapeutic procedures and technologies to reduce costs and improve outcomes. This evaluation of procedures and technologies includes consideration of costs, risks, and benefits for each plan of care. Nurses also have a responsibility to be knowledgeable about principles of financial management, including understanding the costs associated with patient care, the reality of scarce resources in health care, and the need for cost control and cost efficiency.

The graduate-level specialty nurse or advanced practice registered nurse (APRN) is accountable for monitoring resource utilization across settings for patient care and for evaluating cost efficiency in the delivery of nursing care. The graduate-specialty nurse or APRN, specifically the nurse manager and executive, has additional resource utilization responsibility for financial management of departments, organizations, and systems of care, including personnel, equipment and supplies, technology, and physical design.

Application of the Standard in Practice

Education

Nurse educators have a responsibility to teach nursing students at all levels about their obligation to and accountability for resource utilization. Vital to this education is teaching nurses to be critical thinkers about the full patient care continuum. As nurses approach the work of nursing, they use the nursing process. The nursing process should also be used to assess, diagnose, set outcomes, and plan and evaluate resource utilization as it relates not only to the individual patient but also to the unit, department, and system. This approach is particularly important as students learn about their daily care coordination and management responsibilities. However, additional attention must be given to educating the nurse about the realities and drivers of resource utilization for the healthcare consumers and their families and caregivers. This education must also include identification of resources available to the consumer, including insurance and financial sources, healthcare provider and community resources, and innovative therapeutic and technological resources.

Current nursing education stresses the use of evidence to inform practice and to develop an evidence-based practice to be effective and efficient. This is important not only for care of the individual or populations of patients but also for appropriate resource utilization. The plan of care exercise that many nursing students are required to submit should include not only a section on resource utilization for the patient but also an evaluation of the unit.

Administration

In health care today, the challenge is to try to do more with less. Nurse administrators coordinate, direct, and monitor the quality and cost-effectiveness of healthcare resource utilization in their organization—both personnel and patient care. The administrator must partner with the management staff to ensure the availability of adequate resources for patient care delivery (Dunham-Taylor & Pinczek, 2006). In addition, a goal of nursing administration is to value the human resource utilization by assisting nurses to identify and manage their work demands. The administrator needs to facilitate a culture where nurses are involved in those processes and are accountable for appropriate resource utilization. Use of critical pathways is a good example of how nurses can be involved in designing and evaluating resource utilization. A critical pathway is an interprofessional plan of care designed to implement a clinical practice guideline or specific protocol. The pathway provides a plan of care for the specific diagnosis, including all resources that will be used, and for each day or stage of a patient's treatment. The pathway includes key goals and outcomes of care for the specific time frame.

Performance and Quality Improvement

Quality improvement efforts are challenged in resourced-constrained environments. However, as quality efforts within health care continue to question how care is delivered, resource utilization must be a part of the equation. Attempting to balance quality care and appropriate use of resources is an everyday part of the work of nursing. The standard of safe, effective, and financially responsible nursing care demands that nurses participate in identifying waste, redundancy, errors, and inefficient and unsafe systems. However, nurses' involvement in quality improvement for resource utilization must go further. They need to be a part of designing and evaluating the solutions to create safer, higher quality, and more efficient systems. Critical pathways, discussed earlier, can be part of the evaluation of the system of care for a particular patient diagnosis or population of care.

Research

There are several areas for research to evaluate resource utilization in nursing. The first area is the ongoing point-of-care evaluation of the use of resources, including staffing, care coordination, patient throughput, length of stay, and cost of care. Both the research about innovative models of care that balance quality with cost-efficiency and the use of resources and of nursing's role and contribution to care in those models are needed now more than ever. Naylor's transitional care model is one example (see Naylor, Brooten, Campbell, Maislin, McCauley, & Schwartz, 2004; Naylor, Aiken, Kurtzman, Olds, & Hirschman, 2011). The transitional care model provides effective, comprehensive, and evidence-based in-hospital planning and home follow-up for chronically ill, high-risk, older adults. The transitional care nurse is pivotal to this model as is the appropriate identification and use of resources with emphasis on healthcare consumer and family caregiver needs and transition to appropriate community providers and services (Bogner, Miller, de Vries, Chhatre, & Jayadevappa, 2010).

Most recently, attention has been directed at another innovative model of delivery of health care, the patient-centered medical home (PCMH). The evaluation of the cost-effectiveness of this model of care and of how nurses at all levels participate in the PCMH is necessary (IOM, 2011; Baker & Bielsel, 2010; Scudder, 2011).

Conclusion

Standard 15 Resource Utilization describes the expectation that the RN will use appropriate resources to plan and provide nursing services that are safe, effective, and financially responsible. The provision of quality care includes not only appropriately using the nursing process but also accessing resources and assisting the healthcare consumer to navigate resources for care across the continuum. Goals of safe, timely, effective, efficient, equitable, and patient-centered health care are paramount to competent resource utilization in health care.

Case Study and Discussion Topics

Case Study

Medical System X Quality of Care Council members have reviewed outcomes of care and re-admission data for their congestive heart failure (CHF) population. The council has determined that the system is not meeting benchmarks for clinical and process outcomes. In addition, CHF patient re-admissions rates are above both the average national and the average state rates. A task force has been charged to design a program of care across the continuum to better manage CHF patients. The charge includes managing care and accessing appropriate resources at each transition point to have a positive influence on the effectiveness of care and the efficiency of resources for the system, including personnel and use of technology. You are the chairperson of this task force.

Discussion Topics: Initial

1. Whom will you invite to participate?

2. What are the goals, objectives, and activities of this care management program?

3. What outcomes will you measure and why?

Discussion Topics: Follow-Up

1. What methods of resource utilization did the task force use to design this program?

2. What skills and knowledge in resource utilization are important for direct nursing practice?

3. What skills and knowledge in resource utilization are important for managing nursing resources?

4. What are the pros and cons of resource-driven versus outcome-driven models of nursing care delivery?

5. What moral or ethical principles are related to resource utilization in health care?

References and Other Sources

Baker, C., & Beilsel, M. (2010). Evolution of the chronic care role for RNs: Patient-centered medical home. *Nursing Economics, 28*(6), 409–414.

Bogner, H. R., Miller, S. D., de Vries, H. F., Chhatre, S., & Jayadevappa, R. (2010). Assessment of cost and health resource utilization for elderly patients with heart failure and diabetes mellitus. *Journal of Cardiac Failure, 16*(6), 454–60.

Center for Medicare and Medicaid Services. (2012). Overview of accountable care organizations. Retrieved from https://www.cms.gov/ACO/

The Essential Guide to Nursing Practice

Commission for Case Manager Certification. (2011). Definition and philosophy of case management. Retrieved from http://www.ccmcertification.org

Dunham-Taylor, J., & Pinczek, J. (2006). *Financial management for nurse managers*. Burlington, MA: Jones & Bartlett Publishers International.

Gold, J. (2011, October 11). FAQs on accountable care organizations, explained. *Kaiser Health News*. Retrieved from http://www.kaiserhealthnews.org/stories/2011/january/13/aco-accountable-care-organization-faq.aspx

Institute of Medicine (IOM). (2001). *Crossing the quality chasm: A new health report for the 21st century*. Washington, DC: National Academies Press.

Institute of Medicine (IOM). (2011). *The future of nursing: Leading change, advancing health*. Washington, DC: National Academies Press. Retrieved from http://thefutureofnursing.org/resource/detail/patient-centered-medical-home

Naylor, M. D., Aiken, L. H., Kurtzman, E. T., Olds, D. M., & Hirschman, K. B. (2011). The care span: The importance of transitional care in achieving health reform. *Health Affairs, 30*(4), 746–754.

Naylor, M., Brooten, D., Campbell, R., Maislin, G., McCauley, K., & Schwartz, J. (2004). Transitional care of older adults hospitalized with heart failure: A randomized, controlled trial. *Journal of American Geriatric Society, 52*, 675–684.

Scudder, L. (2011, May 27). Nurse-led medical homes: Current status and future plans. *Medscape News Today*. Retrieved from http://www.medscape.com/viewarticle/743197

CHAPTER 19
Standard 16. Environmental Health

Karen Ballard, RN, MA, FAAN

Standard 16. Environmental Health. **The registered nurse practices in an environmentally safe and healthy manner.**

Definition and Explanation of the Standard

In 1995, Lillian Mood, an early nurse environmental health activist, observed that environmental health was "a good fit with the values of the nursing profession regarding disease prevention and social justice" (Mood, 1995, p. vii). This observation underscores the critical role that nurses have played and continue to play in assessing and addressing health issues associated with the cleanliness and healthiness of the environment for their patients, themselves, and others in their workplaces. The American Nurses Association (ANA) considers environmental health, as adapted from the World Health Organization (WHO, 1992), to embrace "those aspects of human health, including quality of life, that are determined by physical, chemical, biological, social, and psychological problems in the environment and also refers to the theory and practice of assessing, correcting, controlling, and preventing those factors in the environment that can potentially affect the health of present and future generations" (ANA, 2010, p. 65). The environment in which a registered nurse (RN) practices includes the "surrounding context, milieu, conditions, or atmosphere" (ANA, 2010, p. 64).

In her *First Rule of Nursing*, Florence Nightingale (1859) cautioned nurses to "[k]eep the air within as pure as the air without." The International Council of Nurses (ICN, 1992, p. 1) has observed that

> *the concern of nurses is for people's health—its promotion, its mainte-nance, its restoration. The healthy lives of people depend ultimately on the health of Planet Earth—its soil, its water, its oceans, its atmosphere, its biological diversity—all of the elements which constitute people's natural environment. By extension, therefore, nurses need to be concerned with the promotion, maintenance, and restoration of health of the natural environment, particularly with the pollution, degradation, and destruc-tion of that environment being caused by human activities.*

Both ANA and ICN have stressed the vital roles that nurses can play in reducing the ecological footprint of the healthcare industry and in mitigat-ing the impact of the disposal of medical wastes including pharmaceuticals on communities and the global environment (ANA, 2004a, 2004b, 2006; ICN, 2002, 2010).

The competencies for Standard 16 are based on ANA's *Principles of Environmental Health for Nursing Practice with Implementation Strategies* (ANA, 2007).

- Knowledge of environmental health concepts is essential to nursing practice.

- The Precautionary Principle guides nurses in their practice to use products and practices that do not harm human health or the environ-ment and to take preventive action in the face of uncertainty.

- Nurses have a right to work in an environment that is safe and healthy.

- Healthy environments are sustained through multidisciplinary collaboration.

- Choices of materials, products, technology, and practices in the envi-ronment that affect nursing practice are based on the best evidence available.

- Approaches to promoting a healthy environment respect the diverse values, beliefs, cultures, and circumstances of patients and their families.

- Nurses participate in assessing the quality of the environment in which they practice and live.

- Nurses, other healthcare workers, patients, and communities have the right to know relevant and timely information about the potentially harmful products, chemicals, pollutants, and hazards to which they are exposed.

- Nurses participate in research of best practices that promote a safe and healthy environment.

- Nurses must be supported in advocating for and implementing environmental health principles in nursing practice.

There is increasing scientific evidence about the association between environmental exposures to heavy metals, pesticides, air and water pollution, and other environmental toxins and about a wide array of health outcomes, including reproductive and developmental problems; cancer; neurological, immunological, and metabolic disorders; and asthma and other respiratory illnesses (EWG, 2005, 2007, 2008, 2009). The current chemical burden experienced by individuals is unprecedented in human history (Goldman & Koduru, 2000). It is also recognized that several environmentally influenced health problems are on a steep rise in the United States: autism, asthma, obesity, certain childhood cancers, and infertility.

RNs handle many different therapeutic chemicals and drugs with differing side effects and exposure rates in the course of their practice. In addition, nurses can experience health reactions to diverse, chronic workplace exposures to hazardous cleaning, disinfecting, and sterilizing agents; radiation; mercury; and other chemicals (EWG, 2007). In one study of physicians and nurses, 18 of the same chemicals were detected in every single participant; all 20 participants had at least five of the six major types of chemicals tested; 13 participants tested positive for all six of these major chemical types; and all participants had bisphenol-A, phthalates, polybrominated diphenylethers (PBDEs), and perfluorocarbons (PFCs)—priority chemicals for regulation by the U.S. Environmental Protection Agency (EPA) and associated with chronic illness, such as cancer and endocrine malfunction (PSR, 2009).

Nurses have an immense capacity to affect environmental conditions for their patients, themselves, and their communities. In addition to their work in reducing harmful chemical, biological, and radiological exposures, nurses can improve the public's health by promoting positive workplace and community environments. Nurses can advocate for green spaces and walkable communities, safe and healthy buildings, and use of environmentally preferable products.

Application of the Standard in Practice

Education

Concerning health and illness, all nurses need to acquire basic knowledge of scientific environmental health concepts, including the basic mechanisms and pathways of exposure to environmental hazards; the prevention and control strategies; and the interrelationships of individuals, communities, populations, and the environment, including the workplace. This knowledge includes assessing the practice environment for factors—such as sound, odor, noise, and light—that threaten health and never serving as a "transfer agent" for the transmittal of infectious materials from the healthcare facility to one's home and community.

Nurse educators must incorporate environmental concepts, principles, and competencies in both basic and advanced curricula across the learning continuum. A single class or course is not sufficient to meet this critical learning need. Curricula must include basic principles of toxicology; disease-specific and toxic-specific information; information on environmental risks in the home, healthcare facility, community, and workplace; methods for environmental and occupational history taking; and ways to expand the nursing process to include the environment as a separate and important domain in assessment. Additional content is needed about the following:

- The use of the Centers for Disease Control's (CDC's) IPREPARE approach for individuals and families.

- The use of the Precautionary Principle and ANA's *Principles of Environmental Health for Nursing Practice with Implementation Strategies* (ANA, 2007).

- The role of federal, state, and local governments in addressing environmental issues.

- The use of environmental research.

- The effects of single-hit, cumulative, and multiple exposures across the lifespan.

- The right to know about one's exposure to potentially harmful products, chemicals, pollutants, and hazards in the home, community, and workplace.

- The professional organizations and advocacy groups that address environmental issues. (Sattler & Lipscomb, 2003)

ANA's *Principles of Environmental Health for Nursing Practice* recommends that all nurses be able to complete an environmental health history; to recognize potential environmental hazards and sentinel illnesses; to make appropriate referrals for conditions with probable environmental etiologies; to access and provide information to colleagues, patients, and communities; and to locate and use referral sources (ANA, 2007). Nurses need to understand their roles as advocates and lobbyists in communicating the potential adverse effects of the environment on health and in developing legislation and regulations to protect the health of individuals and communities. As lifelong learners, RNs can supplement their formal education by becoming environmental health activists through such activities in their practice settings, homes, and communities as they determine the probability of risk, hazard identification, dose response evaluation, exposure assessment, and risk characterizations and as they design risk management plans (ANA, 2007).

Administration

Nurses have a right to work in an environment that is safe and healthy (ANA, 2007). Nurse administrators, chief executive officers, and owners and boards of directors of healthcare agencies and facilities must create an organizational culture that recognizes and supports the incorporation of environmental health principles into nursing practice and advocacy in the workplace. Healthy work environments have been described as workplaces that are supportive of the whole human being, are patient-focused, and are joyful (Shirey, 2006; Ives Erickson, 2010). Nurse administrators can implement as organizational policy the Precautionary Principle, which promotes the belief that "when an activity raises threats of harm to human health or the environment, precautionary measures should be taken even if some cause-and-effect relationships are not fully established scientifically" (Science and Environmental Health Network, 1998).

All employers should expect and assist the nursing staff in being actively involved in identifying and changing hazardous environmental conditions affecting the health of patients, all staff members, and their communities. On a regular basis, they must be supported in communicating about environmental health risks and about exposure reduction strategies. This commitment of administration to an environmentally healthier and safer workplace must be an identified standard of practice for the facility, starting with an employee's orientation and then being expressed as an expectation of all employees in job descriptions and in ongoing performance appraisals.

According to the Planetree, a nonprofit organization, "designs for healthcare settings that address all the human senses and support the patient's mind, body, and spirit provide the basis for a healing environment" (Montague, Blietz, & Kachur, 2009). This approach includes the need:

- to control for sound reduction of excessive noise that interferes with patients' rest and sleep requirements;

- to monitor vital signs and immune system responses; and

- to reduce staff fatigue, stress, and burnout.

The current technical brief on acoustic environment by *Green Guide for Health Care* (2007) provides administrators with suggestions for lowering noise levels and for improving patient outcomes and staff performance levels by reducing intrusive noises from sources such as exterior and mechanical sounds, medical equipment beeps and alarms, building vibration, pagers and overhead call systems, and verbal communication among staff members.

Healthcare facilities can improve the health of their staff members and communities by sponsoring green markets or farmers' markets that encourage the use of locally grown products at affordable prices with demonstrations of simple and effective ways of incorporating them into the family's diet. In addition, there must be a commitment by employers to "green" meetings and work settings that focus on reducing and recycling paperwork and on using products that are as environmentally responsible as possible. The entire facility can become a "multidisciplinary green team."

Performance and Quality Improvement

Increasingly, healthcare facilities are identifying the effects of medical and nursing practices on the outcomes of patient care. There are various accrediting and regulatory agencies and groups at the federal, state, and local levels that establish standards for exposure to environmental hazards; unfortunately, those standards are often not enforceable. Some of the standards-setting groups include the CDC, the National Institute for Occupational Health and Safety (NIOSH), the Occupational Health and Safety Administration (OSHA) through its General Duty Clause, the EPA, The Joint Commission through its Environment of Care Standard, and the Emergency Care Research Institute (ECRI) through its medical device safety reporting and hazard information. Through quality assurance and improvement programs, environmental hazards for patients and staff can be identified and exposure reduction strategies can be developed and implemented.

Research

Evidenced-based practice is central to the nursing profession. Nurses must be able to interpret and use research findings that expose environmental hazards, improve the human condition, and maintain safe and healthy workplaces and communities. Under NIOSH, the National Occupational Research Agenda (NORA) is a partnership program to stimulate innovative research and improved workplace practices and to identify the most critical issues in workplace safety and health. Nurses need to participate in studies that identify the body burden of chemicals that have been acquired during the practice of the profession (PSR, 2009). Other environmental agencies and health activist groups provide information guides and alternative lists on the use of mercury and other chemicals, electronics, pesticides, operating room gases, cleaning products, pesticides, and fragrances in healthcare settings. Nurses must use research findings to "make recommendations for the purchase and use of pharmaceuticals, materials, products, and technology that have been shown to minimize harm to the environment and risk to patients and personnel (ANA, 2007). Most important, nurses need to remember that, when in doubt about the potential risks of healthcare products, they should use the Precautionary Principle before risking harm to patients, staff members, and the environment.

Conclusion

All healthcare workers are responsible for protecting the healthcare environment. As Standard 16 states, nurses need to practice in an environmentally safe and healthy manner. Evidence shows that there is a direct connection between nursing actions and the health of the environment in healthcare agencies. Nurses have the responsibility (1) to become informed about the importance of a healthy work environment and the effect of the environment on health and illness and (2) to use evidence for environmental health in their practices.

Case Studies and Discussion Topics

Case Study 1. Workplace Noise

Nurses understand the effect of a healthy environment on their patients. Health Care Without Harm, an international coalition working around the planet to reduce the ecological footprint of the healthcare industry, sponsors The Luminary Project (TLP), a web site that chronicles the stories of nurses as environmental health activists. Those nurses' stories are inspiring as they address issues such as reducing noise, recycling batteries, using red bags appropriately, managing and disposing of pharmaceuticals, incorporating environmental health into nursing curriculums, lobbying for environmental policies and legislation, and sponsoring green markets for healthcare facilities and their communities.

Consider the experience of Elodia Mercier, MS, RNC, who is a nurse manager at a large medical center in New York City (TLP, 2006). She identified that patient satisfaction surveys revealed patients were disturbed by loud noises on the units, especially at night when they were trying to sleep but also during the day. Nursing staff members indicated that they were bothered by the constant din, but they assumed the noise was inevitable on busy patient care units. The solution was to bring back the "quiet zone" that had been instituted more than 100 years ago by Florence Nightingale.

The staff members knew that they could not eliminate all noise. Their goal was to reduce the overall noise level so that essential sounds, such as those coming from the ventilators and IV pumps, were apparent, yet the atmosphere was quieter for the patients. This goal required changing the work habits of staff members and changing the types of technology being used. A hospital-wide program, Silent Hospitals Help Healing or SHHH, was instituted.

Discussion Topics

1. What steps might you use to explore where and how the problem occurred?

2. Can you describe the environmental problem?

3. What are the underlying causes?

4. How do you propose to resolve the problem?

5. How would you know if you improved the environmental problem?

6. What outcomes would you identify to measure improvement?

Example for Solution and Discussion

Nurses and other staff members had to agree to noise reduction as a goal. Staff members met and were encouraged to identify the "troublesome noises" in the hospital. Some of the changes that were implemented included the following:

- Replace a banging pill crusher that sounded like hammering nails with a pill grinder that was quieter and more cost-effective.

The Essential Guide to Nursing Practice

- Send carts that sounded like subway trains with squealing wheels to the engineering department for overhauls.

- Ask staff members to stop yelling in the hallways, banging closet and cabinet doors, and wearing clogs or other noisy footwear.

- Ask staff members who used beepers, including physicians, to keep them on vibrate.

- Have nurses increase their nursing rounds to see patients more often, thus reducing the use of call bells.

The results were dramatic. Before SHHH, noise levels in the hospital during a typical day were 70–80 decibels as measured on a Type 2 Sound Decibel Meter. During change of shift, those levels could reach 113. For comparison, the sound level of a train or motorcycle is 95 decibels; in a library, it's 55. After the program was implemented, the noise levels in the hospital throughout the day were reduced to the 50-60 decibel range. Finally, SHHH buttons were developed and distributed to patients and staff members, and posters were placed on entrance walls and near hospital elevators, where even visitors noticed and were observed "shhhing" one another.

Case Study 2. A Unit Green Team

Another story on The Luminary Project site is that of Mary Frances D. Pate, DSN, RN, and the nursing staff of the pediatric intensive care unit (PICU) at Oregon Health and Science University. Staff members were concerned that some of their practices might be having detrimental effects on the environment (TLP, 2007). It seemed counterintuitive that, as nurses, they might be healing and causing harm at the same time.

Their environmental efforts began after a sales representative gave them a choice between disposable and reusable oximetery probes and informed them that the used, disposable probes could be returned in a pre-addressed shipping box so the hospital could receive credit for each returned probe. This change led to the formation of the unit's Green Team.

Discussion Topics

1. What steps might you explore to explore where and how the problem occurred?

2. Can you describe the environmental problem?

3. What are the underlying causes?

4. How do you propose to resolve the problem?

5. How would you know if you improved the environmental problem?

6. What outcomes would you identify to measure?

Example for Solution and Discussion

Working with the hospital's recycling program and its environmental health and radiation safety department, the Green Team developed a plan that stressed the importance of keeping trash out of the regulated medical waste bags. Recycling bins were placed where both staff members and patients' families could deposit cans, paper, glass, and plastic. Other actions included the following:

- A graduate student made posters with pictures of the disposables on each bin so families could easily participate.

- Nursing staff members recycled the plastic wrap that encased the unit's linen when it arrived, placed recycling bins for x-rays next to the viewing boxes so the silver in the x-rays could be reclaimed, relocated the battery recycling bin to the front desk where pager batteries are changed, and worked with other hospital departments to find alternatives to mercury-containing equipment and products.

- The PICU nursing staff also hosted a mercury thermometer exchange for all Oregon Health and Science University employees, volunteers, and students.

As a result of the Green Team's work, the PICU received a BRAG award (Business Recycling Awards Group), one of only 400 groups out of 40,000 in the area to have been honored by the city of Portland, Oregon.

Online Resources

The following organizations offer a variety of online materials about environmental health that are useful for nurses:

- Agency for Toxic Substances and Disease Registry at http://www.atsdr.cdc.gov

- Alliance of Nurses for Healthy Environments (ANHE) at http://e-commons.org/anhe/

- American Nurses Association at http://www.nursingworld.org/ (Environmental Health dropdown menu tab under Workplace Safety tab)

- ANA Center for Occupational and Environmental Health at http:// www.nursingworld.org/MainMenuCategories/WorkplaceSafety

- American Association of Occupational Health Nurses at http://www. aaohn.org

- American Public Health Association at http://www.apha.org

- Commonweal's Collaborative on Health and the Environment (CHE) http://www.healthandenvironment.org

- Environmental Protection Agency (EPA) at http://www.epa.gov

- Green Guide for Health Care (GGHC) at http://www.gghc.org/index.php

- Health Care Without Harm (HCWH) at http://www.noharm.org

- The Luminary Project (TLP) at http://www.theluminaryproject.org

- Centers for Disease Control and Prevention. Regulatory information about and resources for Material Safety Data Sheets (MSDS) at http:// www.cdc.gov/niosh/topics/chemical-safety/

- Occupational Safety and Health Administration (OSHA) at http:// www.osha.gov

- Practice Greenhealth (PGH) at http://www.practicegreenhealth.org

- The Sustainable Hospitals Project at http://www.sustainableproduction .org/proj.shos.abou.php

References and Other Sources

American Nurses Association (ANA). (2003). *American Nurses Association adopts precautionary approach.* Silver Spring, MD: Author.

American Nurses Association (ANA). (2004a). *House of Delegates resolution: Environmental health principles in nursing practice.* Silver Spring, MD: Author.

American Nurses Association (ANA). (2004b). *House of Delegates resolution: Inappropriate use of antimicrobials in agriculture.* Silver Spring, MD: Author.

American Nurses Association (ANA). (2006). *House of Delegates resolution: Nursing practice, chemical exposures and right to know.* Silver Spring, MD: Author.

American Nurses Association (ANA). (2007). *Principles of environmental health for nursing practice with implementation strategies.* Silver Spring, MD: Nursesbooks.org. Available from http://www.nursingworld.org/MainMenuCategories/WorkplaceSafety/Environmental-Health/ANAResources/ANAsPrinciplesofEnvironmentalHealthforNursing Practice.pd

American Nurses Association (ANA). (2010). *Nursing: Scope and standards of practice* (2nd ed.). Silver Spring, MD: Nursesbooks.org.

Environmental Working Group (EWG). (2005). *Body burden: The pollution in newborns.* Washington, DC: Author. Retrieved from http://www.ewg.org/reports/bodyburden2/

Environmental Working Group (EWG). (2007). *Nurses' health: A survey on health and chemical exposures.* Washington, DC: Author. Retrieved from http://www.ewg.org/reports/nursesurvey

Environmental Working Group (EWG). (2008). *Pharmaceuticals pollute U.S. tap water.* Washington, DC: Author. Retrieved from http://www.ewg.org/node/26128

Environmental Working Group (EWG). (2009). *232 toxic chemicals in 10 minority babies.* Washington, DC: Author. Retrieved from http://www.ewg.org/minoritycordblood/home

Green Guide for Health Care. (2007). *Green Guide for Health Care: Acoustic environment technical brief.* Retrieved from http://www.acentech.com/resources/Health%20Care%20Acoustic%20Environment%20Technical%20Brief.pdf

Goldman, L. R., & Koduru, S. H. (2000). Chemicals in the environment and developmental toxicity in children: A public health and policy perspective. *Environmental Health Perspectives, 108*(3), S443–S448.

International Council of Nurses (ICN). (1992). *Position on nurses and the natural environment.* Geneva, Switzerland: Author.

International Council of Nurses (ICN). (2002). *Universal access to clean water.* Geneva, Switzerland: Author.

International Council of Nurses (ICN). (2010.) *Health care waste: Role of nurses and nursing*. Geneva, Switzerland: Author.

Ives Erickson, J. (2010). Overview and summary: Promoting healthy work environments: A shared responsibility. *OJIN: The Online Journal of Issues in Nursing*, 15(1).

The Luminary Project (TLP). (2006). Luminary story: Elodia Mercier, MS, RNC. Retrieved from http://www.theluminaryproject.org/story.php?detail=116

The Luminary Project (TLP). (2007). Luminary story: Mary Frances D. Pate, DSN, RN. Retrieved from http://www.theluminaryproject.org/story.php?detail=145

Nightingale, F. (1859/1926). *Notes on nursing: What it is and what it is not*. New York, NY: D. Appleton and Company.

Montague, K. N., Blietz, C. M., & Kachur, M. (2009). Ensuring quieter hospital environments. *American Journal of Nursing*, 109(9), 65–67.

Mood, L. H. (1995). Preface. In *Nursing, health, and the environment: Strengthening the relationship to improve the public's health*. Washington, DC: National Academies Press.

Physicians for Social Responsibility (PSR). (2009). *Toxic chemicals found in doctors and nurses*. Washington, DC: Author. Retrieved from http://www.psr.org/news-events/press-releases/toxic-chemicals-found-in-doctors-and-nurses.html

Sattler, B., & Lipscomb, J. (2003). *Environmental health and nursing practice*. New York, NY: Springer Publishing Company.

Science and Environmental Health Network. (1998). Wingspread Conference on the Precautionary Principle. (January 26, 1998.) Retrieved from http://www.sehn.org/wing.html

Shirey, M. R. (2006). Authentic leaders creating healthy work environments for nursing practice. *American Journal of Critical Care*, 15, 256–267

World Health Organization (WHO). (1992). *Our planet, our health: Report of the WHO Commission on Health and the Environment*. Geneva, Switzerland: Author.

Index

A

AACN. *See* American Association of Critical-
    Care Nurses (AACN)
ABNS. *See* American Board of Nursing
    Specialties (ABNS)
Accountability
    legal regulatory mechanisms and, 6
    quality nursing practice and, 146, 147–148
Accountable care organization
    (ACO), 194
Achievable outcomes, 64
ACO. *See* Accountable care organization
    (ACO)
Administration, application of nursing
    stardards in
    Assessment, 39
    Collaboration, 177–179
    Communication, 157–158
    Diagnosis, 53
    Education, 126–127
    Environmental Health, 205–206
    Ethics, 116–117
    Evaluation, 107–108
    Evidence-based Practice and Research,
        136–137
    Implementation, 97
    Leadership, 167
    Outcomes Identification, 69–70
    Planning, 79
    Professional Practice Evaluation, 189–190
    Quality of Practice, 148
    Resource Utilization, 196
    Standards of Practice and Professional
        Performance in, 28–29

ADN. *See* Associate Degree in Nursing (ADN)
Advanced practice nursing (APN), 128
Advanced Practice Registered Nurse (APRN),
    37, 46, 47, 188
    collaborative competencies of, 175
    EBP skills and, 136
    education competencies for, 124, 125
    leadership competencies of, 165
    levels of planning and, 78–79
    quality nursing practice, 147–148, 149
    resource utilization and, 195
Advanced practice registered nursing, 50–52
Advanced public health nurses (APHN), 53
Agency for Healthcare Research and Quality
    (AHRQ), 3, 147
Agency for Toxic Substances and Disease
    Registry, 210
Aggressive communication, 154
Ahrens, Thomas, 40
AHRQ. *See* Agency for Healthcare Research
    and Quality (AHRQ)
Algorithms/decision trees, 51
Alliance of Nurses for Healthy Environments
    (ANHE), 210
American Association of College of
    Osteopathic Medicine, 174
American Association of Colleges of Nursing,
    154, 174
American Association of Colleges of
    Pharmacy, 174
American Association of Critical-Care Nurses
    (AACN), 155
    standards, 16
American Association of Occupational Health
    Nurses, 211

American Board of Nursing Specialties
(ABNS), 126
American Dental Education Association, 174
American Nurses Association (ANA), 6, 147,
157, 211
attributes, 23
environmental health and, 201, 202
nursing standards by, 24
Patient Safety and Quality Initiative by, 64
*Principles for Social Networking and the
Nurse*, 156
publications by, 1, 11, 24
recognition of specialty, 32
Scope and Standards of Nursing of, 15, 17
scope of practice statement by, 11, 13
social contract and, 3–4
American Nurses Credentialing Center
(ANCC), 29, 126
Magnet Recognition Program®, 16, 17, 29,
69–70, 70, 79, 108, 147
American Public Health Association, 211
ANA. *See* American Nurses Association (ANA)
*ANA Nursing Administration: Scope and
Standards of Practice*, 29
ANCC. *See* American Nurses Credentialing
Center (ANCC)
APHN. *See* Advanced public health nurses
(APHN)
APN. *See* Advanced practice nursing (APN)
APRN. *See* Advanced Practice Registered
Nurse (APRN)
Assertive communication, 154
See also Communication in nursing
practice
Assessment in nursing practice, 35–43
applications
administration, 39
education, 38–39
performance improvement, 39–40
quality improvement, 39–40
research, 40–41
definition and explanation of
data collection, 35–37
synthesis, 37–38
Associate Degree in Nursing (ADN), 125
Association of Medical Colleges, 174
Association of Schools of Public Health, 174
Authentic leadership, 165
See also Leadership
Autonomy, 7

B

Bachelor of Science in Nursing (BSN), 125
Batalden, Paul, 108
Berwick, Donald, 108
BSN. *See* Bachelor of Science in Nursing
(BSN)

C

Care Transitions Program®, 180
Carnegie Foundation for the Advancement of
Teaching's study, 115
Case studies and discussion questions
Assessment, 41–43
Collaboration, 181–182
Communication, 160
Diagnosis, 55–58
Education, 129–130
Environmental Health, 207–210
Ethics, 119–120
Evaluation, 110
Evidence-based Practice and Research,
138–141
Implementation, 99–101
Leadership, 169–170
Outcomes Identification, 71–73
Planning, 81–84
Professional Practice Evaluation, 191–192
Quality of practice, 150
Resource Utilization, 197–198
Causation, 31
CCNE. *See* Commission on Collegiate Nursing
Education (CCNE)
CE. *See* Continuing education (CE)
programs
Center for Medicare and Medicaid
Services, 66
Center for Nursing Classification and Clinical
Effectiveness, 89
Center for Occupational and Environmental
Health, of ANA, 211
Centers for Disease Control and
Prevention, 211
Centers for Medicare and Medicaid Services
(CMS), 2–3
CER. *See* Comparative effectiveness
research (CER)
CINAHL. *See* Cumulative Index to Nursing
and Allied Health Literature
(CINAHL)
Clinical Care Classification System, 47
Clinical nurse leader (CNL) programs, 124
Clinical nurse specialists (CNS)
medical diagnoses by, 46, 52–53
Clinical Practice Model (CPM), 17, 18
CMS. *See* Centers for Medicare and Medicaid
Services (CMS)
CNL. *See* Clinical nurse leader (CNL)
programs
CNM. *See* Nurse midwives (CNM)
Cochrane Collaboration, 134
Cochrane Library, 141
Code of Ethics for Nurses, 17, 113–114
*Code of Ethics for Nurses with Interpretive
Statements*, 24, 113

The Essential Guide to Nursing Practice

Collaboration in nursing practice, 4, 173–182
application
administration, 177–179
education, 176–177
performance improvement, 179
quality improvement, 179
research, 179–180
communication and, 178
competencies for, 174–177
definition and explanation, 173–176
equality and, 178–179
interprofessional practice, 174
intraprofessional practice, 174
transitions in, 177–178
See also Communication in nursing practice;
Interprofessional collaborative practice
Collaborative on Health and the Environment
(CHE), 211
Collaborative reasoning, 175
Commission on Collegiate Nursing Education
(CCNE), 27, 106
Communication in nursing practice, 153–160
aggressive, 154
application
administration, 157–158
education, 156–157
performance improvement, 158–159
quality improvement, 158–159
research, 159
assertive, 154
collaborative nursing practice
and, 178
competencies for, 157
definition and explanation, 153–156
disruptive, 157
leadership standard for, 159
strategies to reduce, 158
incivility and, 156–157
Internet and, 155–156
passive, 153
social networking and, 155–156
stress and, 154
studies, 155
styles, 153–154
See also Collaboration in nursing practice
Comparative effectiveness research (CER), 98
Competence/competency(ies), 7, 24–26, 124, 125
collaboration, 174–177
communication, 157
education, 124, 125
environmental health, 202–203
evaluation, 188
leadership, 165–166
in medical diagnosis, 52
outcomes identification, 68
processes, 107

quality nursing practice, 146
See also Advanced Practice Registered
Nurse (APRN); Graduate-level
prepared specialty nurses; Registered
nurse (RN); *specific standards*
Consultation in nursing practice
Implementation, 95
Continuing education (CE) programs, 125, 126
Coordination of care in nursing practice
Implementation, 93
CPM. *See* Clinical Practice Model (CPM)
CRNA. *See* Nurse anesthetists (CRNA)
*Crossing the Quality Chasm: A New Health
System for the 21st Century,* 106,
137, 194
Cumulative Index to Nursing and Allied Health
Literature (CINAHL), 66, 141

D

DARE. *See* Database of Abstracts of Reviews
of Effects (DARE)
Data collection, assessment and, 35–37
Data synthesis
assessment and, 37–38
Database of Abstracts of Reviews of Effects
(DARE), 141
Decision-making, collaborative, 175
Decision trees/algorithms, 51
Diagnosis in nursing practice, 45–58
applications, 52–54
administration, 53
education, 52–53
performance improvement, 53–54
quality improvement, 53–54
research, 54
definition and explanation of, 45–52
differential, 51
process, 48–52
law and regulation, 50
patient-focused care, 48–49
population-focused care, 49
systems of care, 49–50
types of, 46–48
Diagnostic and Statistical Manual of Mental
Disorders (DSM), 47
Disruptive/inappropriate behaviors, 157
leadership standard for, 159
strategies to reduce, 158
See also Communication in nursing
practice
DNP. *See* Doctor of nursing practice (DNP)
degree
Doctor of nursing practice (DNP)
degree, 124
DSM. *See* Diagnostic and Statistical Manual
of Mental Disorders (DSM)
Duty, 31

E

EBP. *See* Evidence-based practice (EBP)
ECRI. *See* Emergency Care Research Institute (ECRI)
Education, application of nursing stardards in, 27–28
   Assessment, 38–39
   Collaboration, 176–177
   Communication, 156–157
   Diagnosis, 52–53
   Education, 125–126
   Environmental Health, 204–205
   Ethics, 115–116
   Evaluation, 106–107
   Evidence-based Practice and Research, 135–136
   Implementation, 97
   Leadership, 166
   Outcomes Identification, 68–69
   Planning, 79
   Professional Practice Evaluation, 188–189
   Quality of Practice, 147–148
   Resource Utilization, 195
Education in nursing practice, 123–130
   application
      administration, 126–127
      education, 125–126
      performance improvement, 127–128
      quality improvement, 127–128
      research, 128
   definition and explanation of, 123–125
Emergency Care Research Institute (ECRI), 206
Empirical Quality Results, 70
Empowerment, dimensions of, 164
   See also Leadership in nursing practice
Environmental health in nursing practice, 201–211
   applications, 204–207
      administration, 205–206
      education, 204–205
      performance improvement, 206
      quality improvement, 206
      research, 207
   competencies for, 202–203
   definition and explanation of, 201–203
   online resources, 210–211
EPA. *See* U.S. Environmental Protection Agency (EPA)
Equality, collaborative nursing practice and, 178–179
Ethics in nursing practice, 113–120
   application
      administration, 116–117
      education, 115–116
      performance improvement, 117–118

      quality improvement, 117–118
      research, 118
   collaborative decision-making and, 175
   definition and explanation of, 113–115
Evaluation in nursing practice, 105–110
   application
      administration, 107–108
      education, 106–107
      performance improvement, 108–109
      quality improvement, 108–109
      research, 109
   definition and explanation of, 105–106
Evidence-based practice (EBP) and research in nursing practice, 40, 133–143, 166, 168, 178
   application
      administration, 136–137
      education, 135–136
      performance improvement, 137
      quality improvement, 137
      research, 137
   definition and explanation of, 133–135
   ethics and, 118
   online resources
      CINAHL, 141
      Cochrane Library, 141
      DARE, 141
      Google Scholar, 141
      JBI, 142
      MEDLINE, 142
      NGC, 142
      PubMed, 142
      SUMSearch, 142–143
      Trip Database, 142
      VHINL database, 143

F

Failure Mode Effect Analysis, 159
First Rule of Nursing, 202
Formal education for nursing, 124
From Novice to Expert, 80
Future of Nursing: Leading Change, Advancing Health, The, 163
Future of Nursing report, of IOM, 12

G

GGHC. *See* Green Guide for Health Care (GGHC)
Google Scholar, 141
Graduate-level prepared specialty nurses, 37, 39, 40, 41, 68, 92, 95, 106, 124, 125, 134, 188
   competencies of, 165, 175
   levels of planning and, 78–79
Green Guide for Health Care, 206
Green Guide for Health Care (GGHC), 211

H

Hall, Richard, 23
Health Care Without Harm (HCWH), 211
Health Insurance Portability and
    Accountability Act (HIPAA), 117
Health teaching and health promotion in
    nursing practice
Implementation, 94
Healthcare Cost and Utilization Project
    databases, 39
Henderson, Virginia, 1, 4
HIPAA. *See* Health Insurance Portability and
    Accountability Act (HIPAA)
Hospital Consumer Assessment of Healthcare
    Providers and Systems (HCAPS), 39
Houle, Cyril, 24
Human responses, in nursing, 5
Hypothesis testing method, 51

I

ICD. *See* International Classification of
    Diseases (ICD)
ICF. *See* International Classification of
    Functioning, Disability, and Health (ICF)
ICN. *See* International Council of Nurses (ICN)
ICNP. *See* International Classification of
    Nursing Practice (ICNP)
IDP. *See* Individualized development plans (IDP)
IHI. *See* Institute for Healthcare Improvement
    (IHI)
Illinois Nurse Practice Act, 15–16
Implementation in nursing practice, 87–101
    application
        administration, 97
        education, 97
        performance improvement, 98–99
        quality improvement, 98–99
        research, 97–98
    consultation, 95
    coordination of care, 93
    definition and explanation of, 87–92
    health teaching and health promotion, 94
    prescriptive authority and treatment, 96
Improvement Science Research Network
    (ISRN), 180
Incivility, 156–157
Includes identification as the first step
    (ISBAR) strategy, 158
Individualized development plans (IDP),
    189–190
Institute for Healthcare Improvement (IHI),
    3, 80, 107, 147
Institute of Medicine (IOM), 12, 80, 106, 124,
    137, 145, 146, 163, 176, 180, 194
Institutional policies and procedures, 16–17
    AACN standards, 16
    CPM (*See* Clinical Practice Model (CPM))

Forces of Magnetism, 17
    Magnet Recognition Program, 16, 29
Institutional review board (IRB)
    QI projects and, 118
International Classification of Diseases
    (ICD), 47
International Classification of Functioning,
    Disability, and Health (ICF), 48
International Classification of Nursing Practice
    (ICNP), 46–47
International Council of Nurses
    (ICN), 202
International Honor Society of
    Nursing, 143
International Nursing Index, 142
Internet, communication and, 155–156
Interpersonal communication (IPC), 153
    See also Communication in nursing practice
Interprofessional collaborative practice, 174, 176
    competencies for, 174–177
    transitions in, 177–178
    See also Collaboration in nursing practice
Interprofessional Education Collaborative
    Expert Panel, 174
Interprofessional Education Collaborative
    (IPEC), 177
IOM. *See* Institute of Medicine (IOM)
IPC. *See* Interpersonal communication (IPC)
IPEC. *See* Interprofessional Education
    Collaborative (IPEC)
IPREPARE approach, 204
IRB. *See* Institutional review board (IRB)
ISBAR. *See* Includes identification as the first
    step (ISBAR) strategy
ISRN. *See* Improvement Science Research
    Network (ISRN)

J

JBI. *See* Joanna Briggs Institute (JBI)
Joanna Briggs Institute (JBI), 107, 142
Just Culture, 116

K

*Keeping Patients Safe: Transforming the Work
    Environment of Nurses*, 145
Knowledge and skills, 5, 7, 12, 16, 24, 26, 29,
    30, 37–38, 49, 54, 67, 89, 91, 95, 99,
    107, 115, 117, 118, 123, 124–125, 126, 127,
    134, 135, 136, 146, 166, 175–176, 179,
    187, 189–190
    competencies for quality nursing practice,
        146, 147
    leadership, 164
    See also Education in nursing practice;
        Evidence-based practice (EBP) and
        research in nursing practice

L

Law and regulation, 50
  See also Regulation, of nursing practice
Leaders: Strategies for Taking Charge, 164
Leadership in nursing practice, 163–170
  application
    administration, 167
    education, 166
    performance improvement, 167–168
    quality improvement, 167–168
    research, 168–169
  authentic, 165
  competencies for, 165–166
  definition and explanation, 163–166
  disruptive/inappropriate behaviors
    and, 159
  quantum, 165
  servant-leadership model, 165
  skills, 164
  theories, 164–165
Legal regulation, of nursing practice, 6–7
  See also Regulation, of nursing practice
Likert scale, 67
Long-term goal/outcomes, 64
  See also Outcomes identification in nursing
    practice

M

*Magnet®: The Next Generation—Nurses
    Making the Difference*, 108
Magnet Model Components, 17
Magnet Recognition Program®, 16, 17, 29,
    69–70, 70, 79, 108, 147, 167, 168
Management skills, 164
  See also Leadership in nursing practice
Master of Science in Nursing (MSN), 125
Material Safety Data Sheets (MSDS), 211
Measurable outcomes, 64
  See also Outcomes identification in nursing
    practice
Medical Subject Headings (MeSH), 142
MEDLINE, 142
MeSH. *See* Medical Subject Headings
    (MeSH)
Model for Improvement, 98
Model of Professional Nursing Practice
    Regulation, 14–19
  institutional policies and procedures (*See*
    Institutional policies and procedures)
  nurse practice acts, 15–16
  self-determination, 17–19
Mood, Lillian, 201
Morality, 114
MSN. *See* Master of Science in
    Nursing (MSN)
Multidisciplinary green team, 206

N

NANDA-I. *See* North American Nursing
    Diagnosis Association International
    (NANDA-I)
National Center for Nursing Quality®
    (NCNQ®), 71
National Council of State Boards of Nursing
    (NCSBN), 78
National Database of Nursing Quality
    Indicators® (NDNQI®), 39, 64, 65, 80,
    108, 109, 147
National Guideline Clearinghouse (NGC), 142
National Institute for Occupational Health
    and Safety (NIOSH), 206, 207
National Institute of Nursing Research
    (NINR), 98
National League for Nursing Accrediting
    Commission (NLNAC), 27, 106–107
National licensure examination (NCLEX), 78
National Occupational Research Agenda
    (NORA), 207
National Organization of Nurse Practitioner
    Faculties (NONPF), 107
National Quality Forum (NQF), 65, 147
NCLEX. *See* National licensure examination
    (NCLEX)
NCNQ®. *See* National Center for Nursing
    Quality® (NCNQ®)
NCSBN. *See* National Council of State Boards
    of Nursing (NCSBN)
NDNQI®. *See* National Database of Nursing
    Quality Indicators® (NDNQI®)
NGC. *See* National Guideline
    Clearinghouse (NGC)
NIC. *See* Nursing Interventions
    Classification (NIC)
Nightingale, Florence, 1, 4, 202
NINR. *See* National Institute of Nursing
    Research (NINR)
NIOSH. *See* National Institute for
    Occupational Health and Safety
    (NIOSH)
NLNAC. *See* National League for Nursing
    Accrediting Commission (NLNAC)
NOC. *See* Nursing Outcomes Classification
    (NOC)
NONPF. *See* National Organization of Nurse
    Practitioner Faculties (NONPF)
NORA. *See* National Occupational Research
    Agenda (NORA)
North American Nursing Diagnosis
    Association International (NANDA-I),
    46, 47, 66
  classification, 69
*Notes on Nursing: What It Is and What It Is
    Not*, 1
NQF. *See* National Quality Forum (NQF)
Nurse anesthetists (CRNA)
  medical diagnoses by, 46, 50

Nurse midwives (CNM)
  in nursing diagnoses, 46, 50
Nurse practice acts, 15–16
Nurse practitioners (NP)
  medical diagnoses by, 46, 50
Nursing
  areas, leadership role in, 2
  characteristics of, 5
  competency (*See* Competence/
    competency(ies))
  defined, 4–5
  practice (*See* Nursing practice)
  as profession, 23–24
  social context of, 1–4
  social policy statement of (*See* Social policy
    statement)
  standards (*See* Standards of Nursing
    Practice)
Nursing: A Social Policy Statement, 1, 4
Nursing: Scope and Standards of Practice, 11,
    24, 25, 26, 145
Nursing actions, 5
Nursing Interventions Classification (NIC), 46,
    47, 66, 69, 76, 89
Nursing Outcomes Classification (NOC), 46,
    47, 66–67, 69, 76
Nursing practice
  characteristics of, 13–14
  competence in, 25–26 (*See also*
    Competence/competency(ies))
  knowledge base for, 5 (*See also* Knowledge
    and skills)
  regulation of (*See* Regulation, of nursing
    practice)
  scope of (*See* Scope of Nursing Practice)
  specialty areas of, 31–32
  standards of (*See* Standards of Nursing
    Practice)
Nursing process
  in clinical setting, 12
  defined, 25
  Standards of Nursing Practice and, 12–13
  See also Standards of Nursing Practice;
    specific standards
Nursing specialty
  ANA recognition of, 32
  practice, 31–32
Nursing's Social Policy Statement, 1
*Nursing's Social Policy Statement: The Essence
  of the Profession*, 1, 4, 7, 24

O

OASIS. *See* Outcome and Assessment
    Information Set (OASIS)
Occupational Health and Safety
    Administration (OSHA), 206, 211

Omaha System, 47, 67–68
OSHA. *See* Occupational Health and Safety
    Administration (OSHA)
Outcome and Assessment Information Set
    (OASIS), 66
Outcomes, 63, 66
  of nursing actions, 5
Outcomes identification in nursing practice,
    63–73
  applications, 68–71
    administration, 69–70
    education, 68–69
    performance improvement, 70
    quality improvement, 70
    research, 70–71
  characteristics of, 68
  competencies for, 68
  definition and explanation of, 63–68
  NOC, 66–67
  Omaha System, 67–68
  structure, process, and outcomes model, 66
  See also Planning in nursing practice

P

PARIHS. *See* Promoting Action on Research
    Implementation in Health Services
    (PARIHS)
Partnership Culture Model, 17
Partnerships, 4
Passive communication, 153
  See also Communication in nursing practice
Patient-centered medical home (PCMH), 197
Patient-focused care, 48–49
Patient Safety and Quality Initiative, by ANA, 64
Pattern matching approach, 50
PCMH. *See* Patient-centered medical home
    (PCMH)
PDSA. *See* Plan-Do-Study-Act (PDSA) cycle
Peer evaluation, 189
Performance appraisal, 127
Performance improvement, application of
    nursing stardards in
  Assessment, 39–40
  Collaboration, 179
  Communication, 158–159
  Diagnosis, 53–54
  Education, 127–128
  Environmental Health, 206
  Ethics, 117–118
  Evaluation, 108–109
  Evidence-based Practice and Research, 137
  Implementation, 98–99
  Leadership, 167–168
  Outcomes Identification, 70
  Planning, 79–80
  Professional Practice Evaluation, 190

Performance improvement, application of
nursing stardards in (*Continued*)
Quality of practice, 148–149
Resource Utilization, 196
Standards of Practice and Professional
Performance in, 29–30
Perioperative Nursing Data Set (PNDS),
46–47
PHN. *See* Public health nursing (PHN)
Plan-Do-Study-Act (PDSA) cycle, 99
Planetree, 206
Planning in nursing practice, 75–84
application
administration, 79
education, 79
performance improvement, 79–80
quality improvement, 79–80
research, 80
definition and explanation of, 75–79
elements, 76
individualized planning, improvement in, 77
reasoning process, 76
strategies, 76
See also Implementation in nursing
practice; Outcomes identification in
nursing practice
PNDS. *See* Perioperative Nursing Data Set
(PNDS)
Population-focused care, 49
Practice Greenhealth (PGH), 211
Precautionary Principle, nurse administrators
and, 205
Prescriptive authority and treatment in
nursing practice
implementation, 96
Principles for Social Networking and the Nurse
(ANA), 156
*Principles of Environmental Health for
Nursing Practice with Implementation
Strategies* (ANA), 202–203, 204, 205
Process, in outcomes identification, 66
Professional career, application of nursing
stardards in
Assessment in nursing practice, 38–40
Diagnosis in nursing practice, 52–54
See also Education, application of nursing
stardards in
Professional Nursing Practice Regulation,
model of, 14–19
Professional practice evaluation in nursing,
187–192
applications, 188–191
administration, 189–190
education, 188–189
performance improvement, 190
quality improvement, 190
research, 190–191
definition and explanation of, 187–188

Professional regulation, 6
See also Regulation, of nursing practice
Professional Role Competence (ANA), 25–26
Promoting Action on Research
Implementation in Health Services
(PARIHS), 137
Public health nursing (PHN), 127
PubMed, 142

Q

QSEN. *See* Quality and Safety Education for
Nurses (QSEN)
Quality and Safety Education for Nurses
(QSEN), 107, 177, 179
Quality improvement, application of nursing
stardards in
Assessment, 39–40
Collaboration, 179
Communication, 158–159
Diagnosis, 53–54
Education, 127–128
Environmental Health, 206
Ethics, 117–118
Evaluation, 108–109
Evidence-based Practice and Research, 137
Implementation, 98–99
Leadership, 167–168
Outcomes Identification, 70
Planning, 79–80
Professional Practice Evaluation, 190
Quality of Practice, 148–149
Resource Utilization, 196
Standards of Practice and Professional
Performance in, 29–30
Quality of practice in nursing, 145–150
application
administration, 148
education, 147–148
performance improvement, 148–149
quality improvement, 148–149
research, 149
competencies for, 146
definition and explanation, 145–147
Quantum leadership, 165
See also Leadership in nursing practice

R

RAP. *See* Resident admission protocols (RAP)
RCA. *See* Root cause analysis (RCA)
Realistic outcomes, 64
See also Outcomes identification in nursing
practice
Registered nurse (RN), 75
communication, 153
education competencies for, 124, 125

The Essential Guide to Nursing Practice

environmental health and, 201, 203
in evaluation process, 187–188, 189
evaluation process competencies, 188
interprofessional collaborative
    competencies, 174–175
leadership competencies, 164, 165–166
in nursing diagnoses, 46, 50
outcomes identification competencies, 68
quality nursing practice, 145, 148–149
resource utilization and, 194–195
scope of practice for, 78
Registry of Nursing Research, 143
Regulation, of nursing practice, 6–7
    legal, 6–7
    professional, 6
    self-regulation, 7
Research, application of nursing stardards in
    Assessment, 40–41
    Collaboration, 179–180
    Communication, 159
    Diagnosis, 54
    Education, 128
    Environmental Health, 207
    Ethics, 118
    Evaluation, 109
    Evidence-based Practice and Research, 137
    Implementation, 98–99
    Leadership, 168–169
    Outcomes Identification, 70–71
    Planning, 80
    Professional Practice Evaluation, 190–191
    Quality of Practice, 149
    Resource Utilization, 196–197
    Standards of Nursing Practice and, 30
    See also Evidence-based practice (EBP) and
        research in nursing practice
Resident admission protocols (RAP), 66
Resource utilization in nursing practice,
    193–198
    application
        administration, 196
        education, 195
        performance improvement, 196
        quality improvement, 196
        research, 196–197
    definition and explanation, 193–195
RN. See Registered nurse (RN)
Robert Wood Johnson Foundation, 107
Root cause analysis (RCA), 107, 159

S

SBAR. See Situation, background, assessment,
    recommendations (SBAR) strategy
Scope and Standards of Nursing, of ANA,
    15, 17

Scope of Nursing Practice, 11–21
    characteristics, 13–14
    Model of Professional Nursing Practice
        Regulation (See Model of Professional
        Nursing Practice Regulation)
    overview of, 11–13
Self-determination, 17–19
Self-evaluation, 189
Self-regulation, 7
Sentinel Event Alert 40, 159
Servant-leadership model, 165
Short-term outcomes, 64
Sigma Theta Tau International, 143
Silence Kills, 155, 159
Silent Treatment, 155, 159
Situation, background, assessment,
    recommendations (SBAR)
    strategy, 158
Skills in nursing practice. See Knowledge and
    skills
SMART outcomes, 63–64, 68, 69
SNOMED CT. See Systematized Nomenclature
    of Medicine—Clinical Terms
    (SNOMED CT)
Social contract, of nursing, 3
    ANA and, 3–4
Social networking, communication and, 155–156
Social policy statement, 1–9
    overview, 1–7
    in practice, use, 7–8
Specific outcomes, 63
Standard of care, 31
Standards for a Healthy Work
    Environment, 157
Standards of Nursing Practice, 23–33
    applications, 26–30
        administration, 28–29
        education, 27–28
        performance improvement, 29–30
        quality improvement, 29–30
        research, 30
    See also Standards of Practice; Standards
        of Professional Nursing Practice;
        Standards of Professional
        Performance
Standards of Practice, 24, 25
    in administration, 28–29
    in nursing education, 27–28
    in performance and quality improvement,
        29–30
Standards of Professional Nursing Practice,
    24–26
Standards of Professional Performance, 24, 25
    in administration, 28–29
    in nursing education, 27–28
    in performance and quality improvement,
        29–30
Stress, communication and, 154

Structure, in outcomes identification, 66
SUMSearch, 142–143
Sustainable Hospitals Project, 211
Systematized Nomenclature of Medicine—
    Clinical Terms (SNOMED CT), 48
Systems of care, 49–50

T

Tactic, 76
Tenets, of professional nursing practice, 13–14
The Future of Nursing: Leading Change,
    Advancing Health, 124
The Joint Commission (TJC), 2–3, 65, 80, 107,
    147, 154, 159, 178, 206
The Luminary Project (TLP), 211
Theory application, in nursing, 5
Time-framed outcomes, 64
    See also Outcomes identification in nursing
    practice
TJC. *See* The Joint Commission (TJC)
Transitions, in interprofessional collaborative
    practice, 177–178
Trip Database, 142

U

U.S. Environmental Protection Agency (EPA),
    203, 206, 211

V

VHINL. *See* Virginia Henderson
    International Nursing Library
    (VHINL) Database
Vibrameter®, 40–41
Violence, workplace, 157
Virginia Henderson International Nursing
    Library (VHINL) Database, 143
Vital Smarts®, 155

W

Work environment
    communication and, strategies
    to improve, 158
Working diagnosis, 51
Workplace violence, ANA standards, 157
Worldviews on Evidence-Based Nursing, 143

The Essential Guide to Nursing Practice